Traumatic Brain Injury

Rehabilitation Medicine Quick Reference

Ralph Buschbacher, MD

Series Editor

Professor, Department of Physical Medicine and Rehabilitation
Indiana University School of Medicine
Indianapolis, Indiana

▓ Spine

Andre N. Panagos

▓ Spinal Cord Injury

Thomas N. Bryce

▓ Traumatic Brain Injury

David X. Cifu and Deborah Caruso

Forthcoming Volumes in the Series

Musculoskeletal, Sports, and Occupational Medicine

Pediatrics

Neuromuscular/EMG

Prosthetics

Stroke

Traumatic Brain Injury

Rehabilitation Medicine Quick Reference

David X. Cifu, MD

Herman J. Flax Professor and Chairman
Department of Physical Medicine and Rehabilitation

Executive Director
Center for Rehabilitation Sciences and Engineering
Virginia Commonwealth University

National Director
Physical Medicine and Rehabilitation Program Office
Veterans Administration Central Office (VACO)
Veterans Health Administration

Chief
Physical Medicine and Rehabilitation Services
Hunter Holmes McGuire VAMC
Richmond, Virginia

Deborah Caruso, MD

Assistant Professor
Department of Physical Medicine and Rehabilitation
Virginia Commonwealth University

Physiatrist
Spinal Cord Injury Service
Hunter Holmes McGuire VAMC
Richmond, Virginia

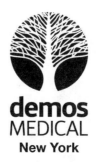

demos
MEDICAL
New York

Acquisitions Editor: Beth Barry
Cover Design: Steve Pisano
Compositor: NewGen North America
Printer: Bang
Visit our website at www.demosmedpub.com

Medicine is an ever-changing science. Research and clinical experience are continually expanding our knowledge, in particular our understanding of proper treatment and drug therapy. The authors, editors, and publisher have made every effort to ensure that all information in this book is in accordance with the state of knowledge at the time of production of the book. Nevertheless, the authors, editors, and publisher are not responsible for errors or omissions or for any consequences from application of the information in this book and make no warranty, express or implied, with respect to the contents of the publication. Every reader should examine carefully the package inserts accompanying each drug and should carefully check whether the dosage schedules mentioned therein or the contraindications stated by the manufacturer differ from the statements made in this book. Such examination is particularly important with drugs that are either rarely used or have been newly released on the market.

Library of Congress Cataloging-in-Publication Data
Cifu, David X.
Traumatic brain injury / David X. Cifu, Deborah Caruso.
    p. ; cm.—(Rehabilitation medicine quick reference)
ISBN 978-1-933864-61-7
 1. Brain—Wounds and injuries—Patients—Rehabilitation—Handbooks, manuals, etc.
I. Caruso, Deborah. II. Title. III. Series: Rehabilitation medicine quick reference.
 [DNLM: 1. Brain Injuries—rehabilitation—Handbooks. WL 39 C569t 2010]
RD594.C55 2010
617.4′810443—dc22   2009050454

Special discounts on bulk quantities of Demos Medical Publishing books are available to corporations, professional associations, pharmaceutical companies, health care organizations, and other qualifying groups. For details, please contact:

Special Sales Department
Demos Medical Publishing
11W. 42nd street
New York, NY 10036
Phone: 800-532-8663 or 212-683-0072
Fax: 212-941-7842
Email: rsantana@demosmedpub.com

Made in the United States of America
10 11 12 13   5 4 3 2 1

To my husband, Chris, who has loved and supported me during my
training and the most challenging aspect of our lives—raising our daughter.
You are my rock, my inspiration, and my best friend.

—D.C.

To my beloved wife, Ingrid, and
cherished daughters, Gabriella and Isabelle, who make it all worthwhile.

—D.X.C.

To all of America's Service Members and Veterans
who remind me every day that "Freedom Is Not Free."

—D.X.C. and D.C.

Contents

Series Foreword xi

Preface xiii

I Traumatic Brain Injury Basics

1. History.. 2

2. Physical Examination.. 4

3. Assessment Scales: Agitation 5

4. Assessment Scales: Balance and Dizziness 6

5. Assessment Scales: Cognition 8

6. Assessment Scales: Concussion Grading 9

7. Assessment Scales: Injury Severity 9

8. Assessment Scales: Level of Arousal and Attention 10

9. Assessment Scales: Orientation 12

10. Assessment Scales: Postconcussion Symptoms 14

11. Assessment Scales: Sleep 16

12. Assessment Scales: Smell 16

13. Diagnostic Tests: Balance and Dizziness 17

14. Diagnostic Tests: Bowel and Bladder Function.......................... 18

15. Diagnostic Tests: Electrophysiologic Evoked Potentials 18

16. Diagnostic Tests: Neuroimaging Findings in Traumatic Brain Injury................ 19

17. Diagnostic Tests: Neuroimaging Techniques.............................. 21

18. Diagnostic Tests: Swallowing 22

19. Diagnostic Tests: Vascular 23

II Conditions

20. Agitation and Restless Behavior.. 26

21. Akinetic Mutism... 28

22. Aphasia, Expressive (Motor).. 30

23. Aphasia, Receptive (Sensory).. 32

24. Attentional Deficits, Mild Traumatic Brain Injury........................ 34

25. Balance Deficits... 36

26. Bladder Issues... 38

27. Bowel Issues 40

28. Central Dysautonomia 42

29. Cognitive Deficits of Traumatic Brain Injury................................ 44

30. Combat-Related Traumatic Brain Injury 46

31. Concussion: Cumulative Mild Traumatic Brain Injury 48

32. Concussion: Mild Traumatic Brain Injury 50

33. Concussion: Postconcussive Symptoms/Syndrome (PCS) 52

34. Concussion: Second Impact Syndrome 54

35. Concussion: Sports 56

36. Coordination Deficits 58

37. Cranial Nerve Deficits—I (Anosmia) 60

38. Cranial Nerve Deficits—V, VII (Face) 62

39. Cranial Nerve Deficits—X, XI, XII (Head and Neck) 64

40. Cranial Nerve Deficits—III, IV, VI (Ocular Muscles) 66

41. Cranial Nerve Deficits—II, VIII, IX (Special Senses) 68

42. Cranial/Skull Defects: Craniotomy/Craniectomy/Cranioplasty 70

43. Deep Venous Thrombosis 72

44. Dementia and Traumatic Brain Injury 74

45. Depression 76

46. Disinhibition 78

47. Dizziness 80

48. Dysarthria 82

49. Dysphagia 84

50. Emotional Lability 86

51. Executive Function Impairment 88

52. Gait (Ambulation) Dysfunction 90

53. Geriatric Traumatic Brain Injury 92

54. Hearing Deficits 94

55. Hemiparesis/Hemiplegia 96

56. Heterotopic Ossification 98

57. Hyperesthesia 100

58. Hypoarousal 102

59. Hypoesthesia/Numbness 104

60. Hypotonia/Flaccidity 106

61. Insomnia 108

62. Locked-in Syndrome 110

63. Minimally Conscious State 112

64. Neglect (Unilateral Spatial Inattention) 114

65. Neuroendocrine Dysfunction: Other 116

66. Neuroendocrine Dysfunction: Syndrome
of Inappropriate Antidiuretic Hormone 118

67. Neurolinguistic Deficits of Traumatic Brain Injury 120

68. Pain: Complex Regional Pain Syndrome 122

69. Pain: General 124

70. Pain: Headaches 126

71. Pediatric Traumatic Brain Injury 128

72. Penetrating Injuries 130

73. Posttraumatic Amnesia 132

74. Posttraumatic Hydrocephalus 134

75. Posttraumatic Seizures 136

76. Posttraumatic Stress Disorder 138

77. Pressure Sores 140

78. Quadriparesis 142

79. Spinal Cord and Traumatic Brain Injury: Dual Disability 144

80. Sexual Dysfunction 146

81. Shaken Baby Syndrome 148

82. Spasticity/Hypertonicity/Rigidity/Clonus 150

83. Tinnitus 152

84. Tremors 154

85. Vegetative State, Persistent 156

86. Vision Deficits 158

87. Visual Perceptual Deficits 160

III Interventions

88. Acute Management of Mild Traumatic Brain Injury 164

89. Acute Management of Moderate to Severe Traumatic Brain Injury 165

90. Agitation: Medications to Treat 166

91. Complementary Alternative Medicine 168

92. Computer-Based Cognitive Therapy 169

93. Constraint-Induced Movement Therapy 170

94. Depression: Medications to Treat 172

95. Disability Determination 173

96. Intensity and Type of Rehabilitation Therapy 174

97. Outcome Assessment and Prediction 175

98. Return to Sports 176

99. Return to Work 177

100. Spasticity: Oral Medications to Treat 178

Index 179

The Rehabilitation Medicine Quick Reference (RMQR) series is dedicated to the busy clinician. While we all strive to keep up with the latest medical knowledge, there are many times when things come up in our daily practices that we need to look up. Even more importantly...look up quickly.

Those aren't the times to do a complete literature search or to read a detailed chapter or review article. We just need to get a quick grasp of a topic that we may not see routinely, or just to refresh our memory. Sometimes a subject comes up that is outside our usual scope of practice, but that may still impact our care. It is for such moments that this series has been created.

Whether you need to quickly look up what a Tarlov cyst is, or you need to read about a neurorehabilitation complication or treatment, RMQR has you covered.

RMQR is designed to include not only the most common problems found in a busy practice but also a lot of the less common ones as well.

I was extremely lucky to have been able to assemble an absolutely fantastic group of editors. They in turn have harnessed an excellent set of authors. So what we have in this series is, I hope and believe, a tremendous reference set to be used often in daily clinical practice. As series editor, I have of course been privy to these books before actual publication. I can tell you that I have already started to rely on them in my clinic—often. They have helped me become more efficient in practice.

Each chapter is organized into succinct facts, presented in a bullet point style. The chapters are set up in the same way throughout all of the volumes in the series, so once you get used to the format, it is incredibly easy to look things up.

And while the focus of the RMQR series is, of course, rehabilitation medicine, the clinical applications are much broader.

I hope that each reader grows to appreciate the RMQR series as much as I have. I congratulate a fine group of editors and authors on creating readable and useful texts.

Ralph Buschbacher, MD

Traumatic brain injury (TBI) and its aftermath have been poorly understood conditions prevalent in human societies for more than 5,000 years. TBI has been an often described and inevitable part of warfare since the sibling rivalry of Cain reportedly caused an uncal herniation in Abel. Evidence of mild TBI has been found in the writings of the Romans and Greeks, in the American Revolutionary and Civil Wars, and in all subsequent wars. While not always well recognized, the short- and long-term effects of postconcussive symptoms have been noted in returning warfighters of all battles. Unfortunately, this also includes the "battles" of a violent society, ranging from child and domestic abuse victims to victims of crime. Brain injury has also been an inevitable result of man's desire to travel faster and farther. From the beginnings of animal-assisted transportation to trains, from bicycles to motorcycles, and from the first Model T to today's hybrid vehicles, the brain's abilities to withstand the superhuman speeds attainable in these devices have been limited. While advances in safety features have enhanced survivability and mitigated many injuries, brain injuries persist. Similarly, despite the enhancements in protective gear and rules, the increasing size, athleticism, and competitive intensity of today's high school, college, and professional athletes have led to an increasing number of brain injuries in sports ranging from football to soccer, from hockey to boxing, and from ice skating to cheerleading. Last, improvements in health care have contributed to the increasing lifespan seen in most nations. While much of this increase has been accompanied by an increase in productivity and physical independence, it has also resulted in an older population with an accompanying higher risk of falling. Brain injuries related to falls in the elderly are the second most common source of emergency room–related TBI. Thus, TBI is not an isolated or unique event for humans but rather a long-standing and pervasive injury with far-reaching consequences.

As the incidence of brain injuries multiplies, heightened awareness of the effects of TBI and the role of early interventions to ameliorate these effects has spawned a desire for practical information to help clinicians provide quality care to TBI patients. A growing number of reference chapters and textbooks have been published that contain comprehensive, academic summaries of TBI and TBI management. These texts serve as excellent sources for academicians, but busy practitioners need a more nuts-and-bolts approach to managing brain injured patients.

This volume has been developed to serve as a user friendly bedside or office tool for the clinician to gain state-of-the-art knowledge and specific, real-world recommendations that will enhance care for the individual with TBI. Each chapter deals with a specific aspect of assessment or treatment. Sufficient background information is provided to allow the practitioner to appreciate the larger context in TBI management. The initial section of the book focuses on the assessment of the individual with acute or chronic sequelae after TBI, from history to physical examination to diagnostic testing. The bulk of the book features alphabetically arranged sections addressing the brain injury conditions and sequelae that will be commonly seen by the academic or community provider. These sections feature a standardized, step-by-step description of how to assess the patient's issues and clinical treatment pearls. There are also red flags and common pitfalls for each problem. All of the information is straightforward, easy to apply, and practical, designed to be implemented by a wide range of clinicians. Specialized areas of TBI care are included for unique patient populations, such as sports or military injury, or sequelae, such as posttraumatic stress disorder or neuroendocrine disorders that may also be seen by some health-care providers. The authors bring a wealth of academic and clinical expertise in brain injury and are active practitioners, so the material in this book comes out of direct experience with TBI patients at every level.

Reader are encouraged to use this volume as a guide to enhance their knowledge and skills. If we can help empower practitioners to expand their clinical service delivery, the multifaceted challenges that individuals with TBI face will be addressed more effectively. There are a growing number of individuals living with TBI-related disability, whether they are the severely disabled from profound injury or the "walking wounded" with potentially life altering sequelae after concussion. All of these individuals deserve and will benefit from expert care and services, especially if these interventions occur in a timely and consistent manner. With this book, we hope to assist in raising the standards of care and ultimate return to productivity and health for anyone who has suffered a traumatic brain injury.

David X. Cifu

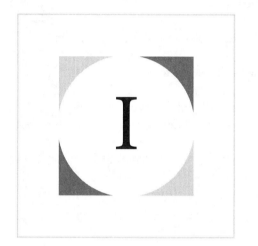

Traumatic Brain Injury Basics

History

Injury Characteristics

Etiology
- Ground-level fall
- Elevated-level fall
- Low-speed motor vehicle collision (< 25 mph)
- High-speed motor vehicle collision (> 25 mph)
- Blunt trauma
- Sports-related
- Military-related (blast)
- Penetrating injury
- Acceleration–Deceleration injury
- "Shaken Baby" injury

Severity
- Alteration or loss of consciousness
- Posttraumatic amnesia
- Computerized tomography scan findings (acute/chronic)
- Magnetic resonance imaging scan findings (acute/chronic)
- Glasgow Coma Score (lowest/best in first 24 h)
- Intracranial pressure readings
- Abnormal brainstem reflex findings

Past Medical History
- Prior traumatic brain injury (TBI)
- History of (H/o) psychiatric illness
- H/o substance/alcohol abuse
- H/o neurologic disorder
- General medical survey
- H/o surgery

Review of Symptoms
- Headaches—frequency, severity, duration, and if they most resemble migraine, tension-type, or cluster headaches
- Dizziness or vertigo—frequency
- Weakness or paralysis—location, severity
- Sleep disturbance—type and frequency, nightmares (associated with posttraumatic stress disorder [PTSD])
- Fatigue—severity
- Mobility—describe limitations
- Balance—describe symptoms and limitations
- Cognitive impairment—severity
  - Memory impairment
  - Slowness of thought
  - Confusion
  - Decreased attention
  - Difficulty concentrating
  - Difficulty understanding directions
  - Difficulty using written language or comprehending written words
  - Delayed reaction time
- Speech difficulties—severity and specific type of problem
  - Aphasia—type, symptoms
  - Dysarthria—type
- Swallowing difficulties—type, severity
- Pain—frequency, severity, duration, location, mediating factors
- Bowel problems—report type and frequency of need for assistance
- Bladder problems—report the type of impairment and the measures needed for maintenance
- Behavioral symptoms severity
  - Anxiety
  - Depression/mood swings
  - Agitation
  - Irritability
  - Restlessness
  - Disinhibition
  - Hypervigilance (associated with PTSD)
  - Paranoid thoughts (associated with PTSD)
- Sexual dysfunction—type
- Sensory changes—location and type
- Visual problems—describe
- Hearing problems—describe
- Decreased smell and/or taste
- Seizures—type and frequency
- Hypersensitivity to sound or light—describe
- Oral and dental problems—describe

Medications

Prescription
- Current
  - All
  - Psychotherapeutics
- Former
  - Used for TBI-related issues

Over the counter
- Current, all

- Former
  - Used for TBI-related issues

Nutraceuticals/supplements
- Current, all
- Former
  - Used for TBI-related issues

Allergies

Social History

Education
- Highest completed level
- Learning disabilities

Productivity
- Current occupation
- Prior occupation
- Disability
- Hobbies

Social supports
- Married/significant other
- Family

Sexuality
- Activity

- Birth control
- Orientation

Functional History

Mobility
- Basic (bed, chair, balance)
- Ambulation (assistive device, distance, safety)
- Community (public transportation, private vehicle)

Activities of daily living
- Basic (grooming, bathing, toileting, dressing)
- Instrumental (cooking, laundry, homemaking, financial management)

Continence
- Bladder
- Bowel

Communication
- Oral
  - Receptive
  - Expressive
- Written
  - Literate

Physical Examination

Cognitive
- Orientation
- Command following (single, multistep)
- Attention
- Concentration
- Memory (short- and long-term)
- Naming/repetition
- Abstract thinking
- Judgment

Behavioral
- Depression
- Anxiety
- Irritability
- Agitation
- Restlessness
- Disinhibition

Musculoskeletal
- Manual muscle (strength) testing
- Joint range of motion (including temporomandibular joint)
- Muscle tone
- Mobility
  - Balance—sitting, standing, dynamic
  - Transfers
  - Gait—indoor, outdoor, stair

Neurologic
- Cranial nerve testing
- Sensory function
- Special sensory
  - Vision
  - Hearing
  - Smell/taste
- Deep tendon reflexes
- Primitive reflexes (frontal release signs)
  - Palmomental reflex
  - Snout reflex
  - Glabellar (tap) reflex
  - Palmar grasp reflex
- Brainstem reflexes
  - Oculocardiac reflex
  - Horizontal oculocephalic/oculovestibular reflex
  - Pupillary light reflex
  - Vertical oculocephalic/oculovestibular reflex
  - Fronto-orbicular reflex
- Bowel/bladder reflexes
  - Cremasteric reflex
  - Bulbocavernosus reflex
  - Anal wink reflex
- Cerebellar testing
  - Finger to nose (upper extremity dysmetria)
  - Heel to shin (lower extremity dysmetria)
- Fine and gross motor coordination (tremor)
- Autonomic nervous system

General Medical Exam
- Skin
- Heart/circulation
- Lung
- Abdomen
  - Digestive
  - Bowel
- Genitourinary
- Endocrine

Assessment Scales: Agitation

Agitated Behavior Scale

- A 0–56-point scale that may be used to measure agitated behavior after brain injury. It may be administered by health care workers at any level of training and family members.

Section I: Traumatic Brain Injury Basics

Agitation Assessment	Score[a]
1. Short attention span, easy distractibility, inability to concentrate.	
2. Impulsive, impatient, low tolerance for pain or frustration.	
3. Uncooperative, resistant to care, demanding.	
4. Violent and or threatening violence toward people or property.	
5. Explosive and/or unpredictable anger.	
6. Rocking, rubbing, moaning or other self-stimulating behavior.	
7. Pulling at tubes, restraints, etc.	
8. Wandering from treatment areas.	
9. Restlessness, pacing, excessive movement.	
10. Repetitive behaviors, motor and/or verbal.	
11. Rapid, loud or excessive talking.	
12. Sudden changes of mood.	
13. Easily initiated or excessive crying and/or laughter.	
14. Self-abusiveness, physical and/or verbal.	

Total Score

No agitation = 14–20; Mild agitation = 21–27; Moderate agitation = 28–34; Severe agitation $\geq$ 35

[a]Key:

1 = absent: the behavior is not present.

2 = present to a slight degree: the behavior is present but does not prevent the conduct of other, contextually appropriate behavior. (The individual may redirect spontaneously, or the continuation of the agitated behavior does not disrupt appropriate behavior.)

3 = present to a moderate degree: the individual needs to be redirected from an agitated to an appropriate behavior, but benefits from such cueing.

4 = present to an extreme degree: the individual is not able to engage in appropriate behavior due to the interference of the agitated behavior, even when external cueing or redirection is provided.

Assessment Scales: Balance and Dizziness

Berg Balance Score

- A 14-item scale used to assess balance for individuals who are able to stand without an assistive device. Each item is scored 0–4, with 0 being the lowest level of functional ability and 4 the highest level of functional ability. It may be used to determine fall risk:
  - 41–56 = low fall risk
  - 21–40 = medium fall risk
  - 0–20 = high fall risk

Berg Balance Score Assessment

Item	Score
1. Sitting to standing	
2. Standing unsupported	
3. Sitting unsupported	
4. Standing to sitting	
5. Transfers	
6. Standing with eyes closed	
7. Standing with feet together	
8. Reaching forward with outstretched arms	
9. Retrieving object from floor	
10. Turning to look behind	
11. Turning 360°	
12. Placing alternative foot on stool	
13. Standing with one foot on stool	
14. Standing on one foot	
Total Score	

Timed Get Up and Go

- The Timed Get Up and Go test records the time required to rise from sitting, ambulate a distance (10 ft), and return to the original seated position without the use of an assistive device. It assesses sit to stand, standing balance, gait, and turning balance.
- Instructions: The person may wear their usual footwear and can use any assistive device they normally use.

Timed Get Up and Go Test

Note: The person should be given one practice trial and then three actual trials. The times from the three actual trials are averaged.

1. Have the person sit in the chair with their back to the chair and their arms resting on the arm rests.
2. Ask the person to stand up from a standard chair and walk a distance of 10 ft (3 m).
3. Have the person turn around, walk back to the chair, and sit down again.
4. Timing begins when the person starts to rise from the chair and ends when he or she returns to the chair and sits down.
5. Record time in seconds.

Categorizing results:
< 10 s = freely mobile
< 20 s = mostly independent
20–29 s = variable mobility
> 20 s = impaired mobility

Computerized posturography

- Computerized posturography is a measure of dynamic balance measured during quiet and challenged standing activities measured on a force plate. Posturography may be performed on an isolated force plate with a computerized screen for visual feedback in a testing laboratory/therapy gym or within the confines of a larger assessment unit (eg, balance master, equitest) that allows for variation to the surrounding visual input (eg, background varied to simulate movement).

Tinnitus Handicap Inventory

- The Tinnitus Handicap Inventory (THI) is a patient questionnaire consisting of 25 questions answered "yes" (4 points), "sometimes" (2 points), or "no" (0 points).

Tinnitus Handicap Inventory

1. Because of your tinnitus, is it difficult to concentrate?	Yes / Sometimes / No
2. Does the loudness of your tinnitus make it difficult for you to hear people?	Yes / Sometimes / No
3. Does your tinnitus make you angry?	Yes / Sometimes / No
4. Does your tinnitus make you feel confused	Yes / Sometimes / No
5. Because of your tinnitus, do you feel desperate?	Yes / Sometimes / No
6. Do you complain a great deal about your tinnitus?	Yes / Sometimes / No
7. Because of your tinnitus, do you have trouble falling to sleep at night?	Yes / Sometimes / No
8. Do you feel that you cannot escape your tinnitus?	Yes / Sometimes / No
9. Does your tinnitus interfere with your ability to enjoy social activities (such as going out to dinner, to the movies)?	Yes / Sometimes / No
10. Because of your tinnitus, do you feel frustrated?	Yes / Sometimes / No
11. Because of your tinnitus, do you feel that you have a terrible disease?	Yes / Sometimes / No
12. Does your tinnitus make it difficult for you to enjoy life?	Yes / Sometimes / No
13. Does your tinnitus interfere with your job or household duties?	Yes / Sometimes / No
14. Because of your tinnitus, do you find that you are often irritable?	Yes / Sometimes / No
15. Because of your tinnitus, is it difficult for you to read?	Yes / Sometimes / No
16. Does your tinnitus make you upset?	Yes / Sometimes / No
17. Do you feel that your tinnitus problem has placed stress on your relationship with members of your family and friends?	Yes / Sometimes / No
18. Do you find it difficult to focus your attention away from your tinnitus and on other things?	Yes / Sometimes / No
19. Do you feel that you have no control over your tinnitus?	Yes / Sometimes / No
20. Because of your tinnitus, do you often feel tired?	Yes / Sometimes / No
21. Because of your tinnitus, do you feel depressed?	Yes / Sometimes / No
22. Does your tinnitus make you feel anxious?	Yes / Sometimes / No
23. Do you feel that you can no longer cope with your tinnitus?	Yes / Sometimes / No
24. Does your tinnitus get worse when you are under stress?	Yes / Sometimes / No
25. Does your tinnitus make you feel insecure?	Yes / Sometimes / No

Score _____

- The THI is graded using the following levels:
  - 0–16 = grade 1 (slight)
  - 18–36 = grade 2 (mild)
  - 38–56 = grade 3 (moderate)
  - 58–76 = grade 4 (severe)
  - 78–100 = grade 5 (catastrophic)

Assessment Scales: Cognition

Rancho Los Amigos Scale, Revised

■ Rancho Los Amigos Scale, revised is a 10-level scale that defines levels of cognitive functioning after brain injury, used to categorize a person's current status.

RLAS Level of Cognitive Functioning

Level I—no response: total assistance

Level II—generalized response: total assistance

Level III—localized response: total assistance

Level IV—confused/agitated: maximal assistance

Level V—confused, inappropriate nonagitated: maximal assistance

Level VI—confused, appropriate: moderate assistance

Level VII—automatic, appropriate: minimal assistance for daily living skills

Level VIII—purposeful, appropriate: stand-by assistance

Level IX—purposeful, appropriate: stand-by assistance on request

Level X—purposeful, appropriate: modified independent

Neuropsychological Testing

■ A standardized cognitive and behavioral evaluation using validated and normed testing performed in a formal environment. Testing uses specifically designed tasks used to measure a psychological function known to be linked to a particular brain structure or pathway. Neuropsychological tests are typically administered to a single person working with an examiner in a quiet office environment, free from distractions. As such, it can be argued that neuropsychological tests at times offer an estimate of a person's peak level of cognitive performance. While neuropsychological testing can be used to identify types and severity of deficits, there is little relationship between specific deficits identified and anatomic (brain)

structures. Typically, individuals who have sustained moderate to severe TBIs have such a wide array of deficits of varying severity that they are unable to fully participate in neuropsychological testing until they have had a period of recovery. As such, only small components of testing may be used to define deficits, and a comprehensive assessment may be delayed until they are being transitioned from an inpatient rehabilitation unit or are looking at resuming some community reintegration (eg, independent living, return to employme nt). While all neuropsychological testing should be individualized based on the expertise of the neuropsychologist and the specific injuries and needs of the patient being evaluated, a standard, brief (1 h) battery that could be used to assess individuals with persistent mild deficits could include:

- California Verbal Learning Test-II—memory measure
- Brief VisuoSpatial Memory Test—memory measure
- Test of Memory Malingering—effort measure
- Wechsler Adult Intelligence Scale IV (WAIS-IV) Working Memory
- Domain score (WAIS-IV): Digit Span, Letter-Number Sequencing, Arithmetic subtests—attention and concentration measure
- Stroop Classic—attention and conc entration measure
- Delis-Kaplan Executive Function System: Controlled Oral Word Association (COWA)—language measure
- WAIS-IV Processing Speed Domain score: Symbol Search, Coding, Cancellation subtests—flexibility and processing measure
- Trail Making Test Versions A & B—attention and concentration measure
- Grooved Pegboard—attention and concentration measure

Assessment Scales: Concussion Grading

Concussion Grading Scales

Source	Grade 1—mild	Grade 2—moderate	Grade 3—severe	Complicated

American Academy of Neurology	No LOC
	   symptoms < 15 min
		No LOC
		   symptoms > 15 min
			+LOC	

Colorado Medical Society	No LOC
	   confusion without amnesia
		No LOC
		   confusion with amnesia
			+LOC	

Cantu	No LOC or PTA < 30 min	LOC < 5 min PTA 30 min–24 h	LOC > 5 min PTA > 24 h	
Williams, Levin, and Eisenberg				Evidence of subarachnoid hemorrhage on initial CT scan

LOC = loss of consciousness; PTA = posttraumatic amnesia; CT = computerized tomography.

Suggested Reading

1. American Academy of Neurology Practice Committee. *Neurology* 1997;48:581–585.
2. Colorado Medical Society. *Report of the Sports Medicine Commitee. Guidelines for the Management of Concussion in Sports.* Colorado Medical Society; 1990 (Revised May 1991). Class III.
3. Cantu RC. Guidelines for return to contact sports after a Cerebral Concussion *Physician Sports Med* 1986;14(10):75–76, 79, 83.
4. Williams D, Levin H, Eisenberg H. Mild head injury classification. *Neurosurg* 1990;27:422–428.

Assessment Scales: Injury Severity

Glasgow Coma Score

■ Glasgow Coma Score is a 3–15 point score that assesses level of consciousness after a brain injury, examining eye opening (1–4), verbalization (1–5), and motor response (1–6). It is the "gold standard" for acute assessment of injury severity and has been useful as a reliable predictor of initial survival and short-term outcome.

Glasgow Coma Scale

	Points					
	1	**2**	**3**	**4**	**5**	**6**
Eyes	Does not open eyes	Opens eyes in response to painful stimuli	Opens eyes in response to voice	Opens eyes spontaneously	N/A	N/A
Verbal	Makes no sounds	Incomprehensible sounds	Utters inappropriate words	Confused, disorientated	Oriented, converses normally	N/A
Motor	Makes no movements	Extension to painful stimuli	Abnormal flexion to painful stimuli	Flexion/ withdrawal to painful stimuli	Localizes painful stimuli	Obeys commands

Mild injury = 13–15; Moderate injury = 9–12; Severe injury = 6–8; Very severe injury = 3–5.

Assessment Scales: Level of Arousal and Attention

Glasgow Coma Score

- Glasgow Coma Score is a 3–15 point score that assesses level of consciousness after a brain injury, examining eye opening (1–4), verbalization (1–5), and motor response (1–6). It is the "gold standard" for acute assessment of injury severity and has been useful as a reliable predictor of initial survival and short-term outcome.

Coma/Near Coma Scale

1. Auditory
    a. Bell ringing
    b. Command responsivity
2. Visual
    a. Light flashes
    b. Follow face and look at me
3. Threat
    a. Move hand to within 1–3 in of eyes
4. Olfactory (occlude tracheostomy 3–5 s)
    a. Ammonia under nose for 2 s
5. Tactile
    a. Shoulder tap
    b. Nasal swab
6. Pain
    a. Pressure on finder nail
    b. Ear pinch
7. Vocalization (spontaneous)

Level 0 = no coma (score = 0.00–0.89)
Level 1 = near coma (score = 0.90–2.00)
Level 2 = moderate coma (score = 2.01–2.89)
Level 3 = marked Coma (score = 2.90–3.49)
Level 4 = extreme coma (score = 3.5–4.00)

Coma/Near Coma Scale

- The Coma/Near Coma (CNC) scale was developed to measure small clinical changes in patients with severe brain injuries who function at very low levels characteristic of near-vegetative and vegetative states. Individuals are tested by at least two independent raters and are tested during a period of "awakeness." The CNC has five levels, based on 11 items, rated 0–4 that can be scored to indicate severity of sensory, perceptual, and primitive response deficits.

JFK Coma Recovery Scale

Domain	Score
Auditory function scale	
4—Consistent movement to command[a]	
3—Reproducible movement to command[a]	
2—Localization to sound	
1—Auditory startle	
0—None	
Visual function scale	
5—Object recognition[a]	
4—Object localization: reaching[a]	
3—Visual pursuit[a]	
2—Fixation[a]	
1—Visual startle	
0—None	
Motor function scale	
6—Functional object use[b]	
5—Automatic motor response[a]	
4—Object manipulation[a]	
3—Localization to noxious stimulation[a]	
2—Flexion withdrawal	
1—Abnormal posturing	
0—None/flaccid	
Oromotor/verbal function scale	
3—Intelligible verbalization[a]	
2—Vocalization/oral movement	
1—Oral reflexive movement	
0—None	
Communication scale	
2—Functional: accurate[b]	
1—Nonfunctional: intentional[a]	
0—None	
Arousal scale	
3—Attention	
2—Eye opening w/o stimulation	
1—Eye opening with stimulation	
0—Unarousable	
Total score	

[a]Denotes minimal conscious state
[b]Denotes emergence from minimal conscious state

JFK Coma Recovery Scale

■ The purpose of the JFK Coma Recovery scale is to assist with the differential diagnosis, prognostic assessment, and treatment planning for patients with disorders of consciousness. The scale consists of six subscales addressing auditory, motor, oromotor, communications, and arousal functions, and ranges 0–23. The subscales are hierarchically arranged with lowest scores representing reflexive activity and the higher scores representing cognitively mediated activities.

Moss Attention Rating Scale

■ The 22-item Moss Attention Rating Scale (MARS) is an observational rating scale that measures attention-related behavior in patients with TBI who have emerged from coma (Rancho Los Amigos Scale of IV or greater). Each of the 22 items is rated on 0–4 point scale, and the total score is converted to a 0–100 point final score. The MARS is useful to monitor progress in therapy and response to specific interventions (eg, medications).

Moss Attention Rating Scale

Please do not leave any items blank. If you are not sure how to answer, just make your best guess.
1 = Definitely false
2 = False, for the most part
3 = Sometimes true, sometimes false
4 = True, for the most part
5 = Definitely true

1. _____ Is restless or fidgety when unoccupied
2. _____ Sustains conversation without interjecting irrelevant or off-topic comments
3. _____ Persists at a task or conversation for several minutes without stopping or "drifting off"
4. _____ Stops performing a task when given something else to do or to think about
5. _____ Misses materials needed for tasks even though they are within sight and reach
6. _____ Performance is best early in the day or after a rest
7. _____ Initiates communication with others
8. _____ Fails to return to a task after an interruption unless prompted to do so
9. _____ Looks toward people approaching
10. _____ Persists with an activity or response after being told to stop
11. _____ Has no difficulty stopping one task or step to begin the next one
12. _____ Attends to nearby conversations rather than the current task or conversation
13. _____ Tends not to initiate tasks that are within his/her capabilities
14. _____ Speed or accuracy deteriorates over several minutes on a task but improves after a break
15. _____ Performance of comparable activities is inconsistent from one day to the next
16. _____ Fails to notice situations affecting current performance, eg, wheelchair hitting against table
17. _____ Perseverates on previous topics of conversation or previous actions
18. _____ Detects errors in his/her own performance
19. _____ Initiates activity (whether appropriate or not) without cuing
20. _____ Reacts to objects being directed toward him/her
21. _____ Performs better on tasks when directions are given slowly
22. _____ Begins to touch or manipulate nearby objects not related to task

Score _____

Assessment Scales: Orientation

Galveston Orientation and Amnesia Test

- Galveston Orientation and Amnesia Test (GOAT) is a 0–100 point scale to assess memory and orientation after brain injury, specifically to determine if an individual has recovered from posttraumatic amnesia (PTA). A score of >70 for three consecutive days is considered the threshold for emergence from PTA. There is a modified GOAT, with choices, for individuals with expressive aphasia, mutism, or severe dysarthria and for those who are intubated (a score of >60 on two consecutive days defines emergence from PTA).

Galveston Orientation and Amnesia Test

Question	Score
1. What is your name? (2 points)	
2. When were you born? (4 points)	
3. Where do you live? (4 points)	
4. Where are you now?	
a. City (5 points)	
b. Hospital (do not need exact name—5 points)	
5. On what date were you admitted to the hospital? (5 points)	
6. How did you get to the hospital? (5 points)	
7. What is the first event you remember after your injury? (5 points)	
8. Can you describe in detail (date, time, companions) the first event you recall after your injury? (5 points)	
9. Can you describe your last event you recall before your injury? (5 points)	
10. Can you describe in detail the last event you recall before your injury? (5 points)	
11. What time is it now? (5 points, remove 1 point for each 30 min incorrect)	
12. What day of the week is it? (5 points, 1 point removed for each wrong day)	
13. What date of the month is it? (5 points, 1 point removed for each date off)	
14. What month is it? (15 points, 5 points removed for each month off)	
15. What year is it? (30 points, 10 points removed for each year off)	
Total score	

Modified GOAT—Provide three choices (one correct) for each question.

Question	Score
1. When were you born? (4 points)	
a. Correct day/month but 5 years earlier than actual date	
b. Correct date	
c. Correct year but different day/month	
2. Where are you now? (city; 5 points)	
a. Correct city	
b. Local city	
c. Local city	

(Continued)

Modified GOAT (Continued)

Question	Score

3. Where are you now? (hospital; 5 points)
   a. School
   b. Hospital
   c. Office

4. On what date were you admitted to the hospital? (5 points)
   a. Correct date
   b. Correct day/year but 1month earlier
   c. One week prior to admission

5. How did you get here? (5 points)
   a. Car
   b. Ambulance
   c. Helicopter

6. What time is it now? (5 points)
   a. Six hours prior to current time
   b. Correct time
   c. Two hours after current time

7. What day of the week is it? (5 points)
   a. Correct day
   b. Two days later
   c. Four days later

8. What date of the month is it? (5 points)
   a. Two days earlier
   b. Correct date
   c. Two days later

9. What month is it? (5 points)
   a. Four months earlier
   b. Two months earlier
   c. Correct month

10. What year is it? (5 points)
   a. Two years earlier
   b. Correct year
   c. Two years later

Total score

Orientation Group Monitoring System

■ The Orientation Group Monitoring System is a reality orientation group for brain injured patients used to improve attentional deficits, confusion, and anterograde amnesia during the period of PTA. Seven behavioral objectives are used to define adequate orientation, attention immediate recall, episodic recall, and the use of memory aides. Daily performance of each of these areas is aggregated to establish a weekly summary score.

Westmead PTA Scale

■ The Westmead PTA Scale is a set of nine cards with seven orientation questions and five memory items designed to objectively measure the period of PTA. A person is determined to be out of PTA when he/she can achieve a perfect score of 12 on the Westmead PTA for three consecutive days.

Assessment Scales: Postconcussion Symptoms

Rivermead Postconcussion Symptoms Questionnaire

■ This questionnaire can be administered to a person who sustains a concussion to measure the severity of 16 different symptoms commonly found after mild traumatic brain injury. The person is ask to rate how severe (0–4) each of the symptoms has been over the past 24 hours compared to how it was before the injury.

Rivermead Postconcussion Symptoms Questionnaire

For each one, please circle the number closest to your answer

0 = not experienced at all
1 = no more of a problem
2 = a mild problem
3 = a moderate problem
4 = a severe problem

Compared with before the accident, do you now (ie, over the last 24 h) suffer from

Headaches	0 1 2 3 4
Feelings of dizziness	0 1 2 3 4
Nausea and/or vomiting	0 1 2 3 4
Noise sensitivity, easily upset by loud noise	0 1 2 3 4
Sleep disturbance	0 1 2 3 4
Fatigue, tiring more easily	0 1 2 3 4
Being irritable, easily angered	0 1 2 3 4
Feeling depressed or tearful	0 1 2 3 4
Feeling frustrated or impatient	0 1 2 3 4
Forgetfulness, poor memory	0 1 2 3 4
Poor concentration	0 1 2 3 4
Taking longer to think	0 1 2 3 4
Blurred vision	0 1 2 3 4
Light sensitivity, Easily upset by bright light	0 1 2 3 4
Double vision	0 1 2 3 4
Restlessness	0 1 2 3 4

Score _____

Neurobehavioral Symptom Inventory

■ The Neurobehavioral Symptom Inventory is a questionnaire that can be administered to a person who sustains a concussion to measure the severity of 22 different symptoms commonly found after mild traumatic brain injury. The person is asked to rate how severe (0–4) each of the symptoms has been compared to how it was before the injury.

Neurobehavioral Symptom Inventory

For each one, please circle the number closest to your answer

None (0) = rarely if ever present; not a problem at all

Mild (1) = occasionally present, but it does not disrupt activities; I can usually continue what I am doing; does not really concern me.

Moderate (2) = often present, occasionally disrupts my activities; I can usually continue what I am doing with some effort; I am somewhat concerned.

Severe (3) = frequently present and disrupts activities; I can only do things that are fairly simple or take little effort; I feel like I need help.

Very severe (4) = almost always present and I have been unable to perform at work, school, or home due to this problem; I probably cannot function without help

Compared with before the accident how have you been doing with the following symptoms

Symptom	None	Mild	Moderate	Severe	Very severe
Feeling dizzy	0	1	2	3	4
Loss of balance	0	1	2	3	4
Poor coordination, clumsy	0	1	2	3	4
Headaches	0	1	2	3	4
Nausea	0	1	2	3	4
Vision problems, blurring, trouble seeing	0	1	2	3	4
Sensitivity to light	0	1	2	3	4
Hearing difficulty	0	1	2	3	4
Sensitivity to noise	0	1	2	3	4
Numbers or tingling on parts of my body	0	1	2	3	4
Change in taste and/or smell	0	1	2	3	4
Loss of appetite or increase appetite	0	1	2	3	4
Poor concentration, cannot pay attention	0	1	2	3	4
Forgetfulness, cannot remember things	0	1	2	3	4
Difficulty making decisions	0	1	2	3	4
Slowed thinking, difficulty getting organized, cannot finish things	0	1	2	3	4
Fatigue, loss of energy, getting tired easily	0	1	2	3	4
Difficulty falling or staying asleep	0	1	2	3	4
Feeling anxious or tense	0	1	2	3	4
Feeling depressed or sad	0	1	2	3	4
Irritability, easily annoyed	0	1	2	3	4
Poor frustration tolerance, feeling easily overwhelmed by things	0	1	2	3	4

Score _____

Assessment Scales: Sleep

Multiple Sleep Latency Test

- The Multiple Sleep Latency Test is a sleep disorder diagnostic tool used to measure the time it takes from the start of a daytime nap period to the first signs of sleep, called "sleep latency." This test measures "sleepiness".

Multiple Sleep Latency Test

Minutes to Sleep	Sleepiness
0–5	Severe
5–10	Troublesome
10–15	Manageable
15–20	Excellent

Epworth Sleepiness Scale

- This is a patient questionnaire used to measure daytime sleepiness, ranked from 0 (no chance of dozing) to 3 (high chance of dozing), in a variety of settings, sitting and reading, sitting inactive in a public place, sitting as a car passenger for an hour, lying down in the afternoon, sitting and talking to someone, sitting quietly after lunch, and sitting in a car stuck in traffic. It is scored as either "average" (0–9) or "recommend referral to a sleep specialist" (10–24).

Epworth Sleepiness Scale

Chance of dozing
0 = no chance of dozing
1 = slight chance of dozing
2 = moderate chance of dozing
3 = high chance of dozing

Situation	Chance of dozing
Sitting and reading	
Watching TV	
Sitting inactive in a public place (eg, a theater or a meeting)	
As a passenger in a car for an hour without a break	
Lying down to rest in the afternoon when circumstances permit	
Sitting and talking to someone	
Sitting quietly after a lunch without alcohol	
In a car, while stopped for a few minutes in traffic	

Score _____

Assessment Scales: Smell

University of Pennsylvania Smell Identification Test

- The University of Pennsylvania Smell Identification Test is a 40-item smell recognition test via scratch and sniff cards. Normal individuals will score in the 30 s (ie, 30 smells detected correctly), individuals with hyposmia in 20 s, and individuals with anosmia with scores closer to 10. The cards also include odors that can be detected via both the olfactory and trigeminal nerves to eliminate malingering.

Diagnostic Tests: Balance and Dizziness

Caloric testing

- Caloric testing is used to measure the functioning of the labyrinthian system of the inner ear. Pupillary findings (eg, horizontal and vertical nystagmus) and subjective reports of vertigo are recorded in response to cold water injected into the ear canals.

Electronystagmography

- Electronystagmography is an electrophysiologic measure of pupillary response to vertical and horizontal visual stimuli.

Dix-Hallpike Maneuver

- Dix-Hallpike maneuver is an assessment of the individual's subjective report of vertigo to rapid movement from sitting to lying with head rotated. Used as an assessment for benign paroxysmal positional vertigo.

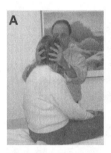 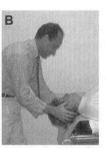 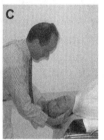
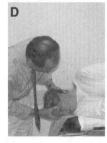 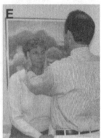

The Canalith Repositioning Maneuver for left-sided benign paroxysmal postural vertigo. (A) The starting position is identical to the initial position in the Dix-Hallpike test, with the cervical spine rotated 45° to the left. (B) The patient is brought into supine, and the cervical spine is extended approximately 10° (45° of left cervical rotation is maintained). (C) The cervical spine is rotated 90° to the right to end up in 45° rotation to the right. (D) The patient is rotated onto their right side, maintaining the cervical rotation to the right. The cervical spine is brought out of extension and is laterally flexed to the right. (E) The patient is brought into sitting. As the patient rises from right side lying to sitting, the cervical rotation to the right is maintained. With permission from Zasler ND, Katz DI, Zafonte RD. *Brain Injury Medicine: Principles and Practice.* New York: Demos Medical Publishing; 2007.

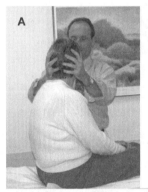 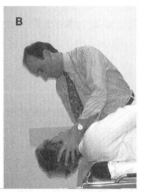

The left Dix-Hallpike Test. (A) The patient sits with legs extended on the table and cervical spine rotated 45° to the left. The examiner places his hands on either side of the patient's head, with his right forearm behind the patient's left shoulder. (B) The patient is quickly brought into supine, and the cervical spine extended approximately 10°. The examiner observes the patient for nystagmus and symptoms. With permission from Zasler ND, Katz DI, Zafonte RD. *Brain Injury Medicine: Principles and Practice.* New York: Demos Medical Publishing; 2007.

Diagnostic Tests: Bowel and Bladder Function

Bowel Manometry
- Bowel manometry is the measurement of pressures within the lower bowel and electrical activity of the internal and external anal sphincters while varying levels of volume are introduced into the bowel. These values are also measured during defecation. These values are used to assess for causes of constipation and incontinence after traumatic brain injury.

Bladder Urodynamics
- Bladder urodynamics is the measurement of pressures within the bladder and electrical activity of the internal and external urinary sphincters during varying levels of volume introduced into the bladder. These values and the rate of flow are also measured during urination. These values are used to assess for causes of urinary retention and incontinence after TBI.

Diagnostic Tests: Electrophysiologic Evoked Potentials

Electroencephalography
- An electroencephalography (EEG) is the recording of electrical activity along the scalp produced by firing of neurons within the brain. An EEG refers to the recording of the brain's spontaneous electrical activity over a short period of time (eg, 20–30 min) and is most commonly used to diagnose and/or localize epileptic activity. EEG may also be used to confirm a diagnosis of coma and encephalopathies.

Brainstem Auditory Evoked Response
- A Brainstem Auditory Evoked Response is a hearing test that detects electrical activity in the cochlea and auditory pathways in the brain. An auditory stimulus is played, and a response waveform is recorded from electrodes placed on the scalp and around the ear. It is particularly useful to assess for deafness in comatose or communication-limited patients.

Visual Evoked Potential
- A Visual Evoked Potential is a vision test using visual stimuli, flashing lights or checkerboards on a visual screen, while an EEG recording is made over the occipital scalp. It is particularly useful to assess for blindness in comatose or communication-limited patients.

Electromyogram
- It is a two-part examination used to assess the integrity of the peripheral nervous and muscular systems. An electromyogram consists of a nerve conduction study to assess the functioning of the peripheral nerves, using electrical stimuli and recording electrodes, and a needle electrical examination to assess the functioning of the neuromuscular junction and skeletal muscle.

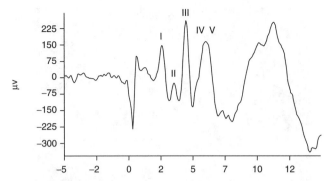

Normal brainstem auditory–evoked potential waveform. (With permission from Zasler ND, Katz DI, Zafonte RD. *Brain Injury Medicine: Principles and Practice.* New York: Demos Medical Publishing; 2007.)

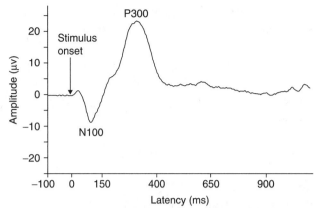

Normal auditory event-related potential waveforms from pure tone (1000 vs 500 Hz) discrimination task. (With permission from Zasler ND, Katz DI, Zafonte RD. *Brain Injury Medicine: Principles and Practice.* New York: Demos Medical Publishing; 2007.)

Section I: Traumatic Brain Injury Basics

Diagnostic Tests: Neuroimaging Findings in Traumatic Brain Injury

Common Neuroimaging Findings after TBI

- Diffuse axonal injury (DAI) describes the microscopic hemorrhage that occurs as a result of acute stretching of white matter tracts after TBI, specifically from acceleration-deceleration injury. DAI is the most common explanation for the acute confusion that occurs in individuals with moderate TBI and the transient alteration of consciousness that occurs in individuals with mild TBI. It is most commonly seen at the gray-white junction of the brain between the cortex and midbrain. DAI may be visualized on acute (i.e., within 7 days of injury) neuroimaging, specifically MRI and the dynamic neuroimaging techniques, such as functional MRI (fMRI), positron emisson tomography (PET) or single photon emisson computed tomography (SPECT).

Subarachnoid Hemorrhage

- Subarachnoid hemorrhage occurs with almost any degree of brain injury, most commonly in the interpeduncular cistern. It is readily visualized on computerized tomography scan. It has little prognostic value, but may predispose patients acute and/or chronic

posttraumatic hydrocephalus if in significant volume (ie, > 50 cc).

Subdural Hematoma

- Subdural hematoma (SDH) occurs with moderate focal skull trauma, particularly in individuals who have pre-existing cerebral atrophy that creates "space" within the skull (eg, older adults) and those on blood thinners. In older adults with significant cerebral atrophy, SDHs may accumulate spontaneously or with minimal trauma, and may go unnoticed for months. While the lentiform-shaped hematomas are easily removed surgically, SDHs are signs of significant underlying brain trauma and may also lead to focal edema. The need for urgent surgical removal of SDHs is a poor prognostic indicator for short- and long-term functional outcome.

Epidural Hematoma

- Epidural hematoma (EDH) occurs with moderate to severe focal skull trauma, usually with accompanying transverse temporal skull fracture. An EDH is a neurosurgical emergency, but when rapidly removed, they rarely result in significant long-term functional sequelae.

Intracerebral Hematoma

■ Intracerebral hematoma or intraparenchymal hematoma is a focal collection of blood within one or more of the lobes of the cerebral cortex, often the result of either direct skull trauma, penetrating injury, or a coup-contracoup injury. These focal injuries are often accompanied by focal functional deficits. Bilateral or multilobe injuries have a higher likelihood of resulting in long-term functional deficits.

Coup-Contracoup Injury

■ Coup-contracoup injury results from the continued movement of the brain within the skull after a moderate to high-speed injury. Most commonly, with a head-on injury, the anterior brain (ie, inferior frontal lobes, anterior temporal lobes) is initially traumatized against the inside of the frontal zone of the skull, and then as the brain rebounds from the impact, the posterior brain (ie, occipital lobes) is traumatized against the inside of the occipital skull. The same biomechanical injury can occur to the right and left sides of the brain with a side impact injury. These injuries will often result in both ICH- and SDH-type injuries.

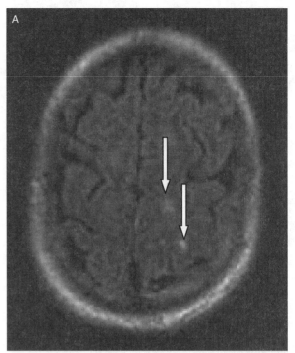

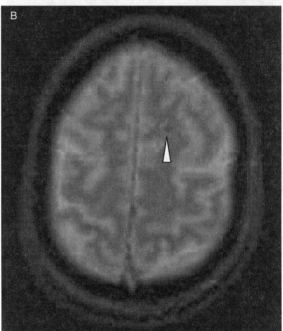

Diffuse axonal injury (DAI): axial FLAIR MRI (A) demonstrates foci of increased signal intensity within the deep bifrontal and left parietal white matter (arrows). Axial gradient echo (B) demonstrates a focus of magnetic susceptibility in the left frontal white matter (arrowhead). These foci are typical of petechial hemorrhages seen in DAI. (With permission from Zasler ND, Katz DI, Zafonte RD. *Brain Injury Medicine: Principles and Practice.* New York: Demos Medical Publishing; 2007.)

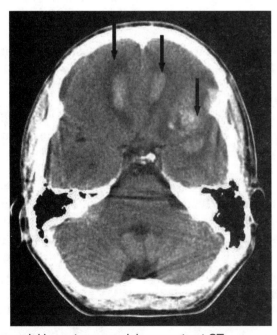

Intra-axial hematomas: axial noncontrast CT demonstrates intra-axial contusions in the bilateral frontal lobes and left temporal lobe (arrows). There is associated vasogenic edema. (With permission from Zasler ND, Katz DI, Zafonte RD. *Brain Injury Medicine: Principles and Practice.* New York: Demos Medical Publishing; 2007.)

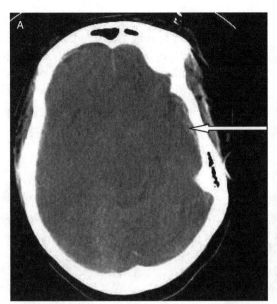 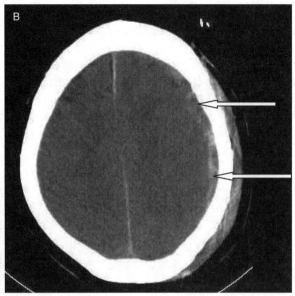

Brain swelling: axial noncontrast CT (A, B) demonstrates a left fronto-parietal subdural hematoma (arrow) and diffuse effacement of sulci and decreased gray/white matter differentiation. These findings are consistent with brain swelling. (With permission from Zasler ND, Katz DI, Zafonte RD. *Brain Injury Medicine: Principles and Practice.* New York: Demos Medical Publishing; 2007.)

Diagnostic Tests: Neuroimaging Techniques

Neuroimaging

■ Radiological testing designed to assess the structure and functional status of the brain and intracranial contents (eg, blood vessels, cerebrospinal fluid). Plain film radiographs visualize the skull but offer limited insights into intracranial structures.

Computerized Tomography

■ Computerized tomography are 360-degree reconstructions of radiographic slices of the brain that are useful to assess for cranial abnormalities, and medium to large intracranial abnormalities, such as intracranial masses and mass effects, bleeding and infection, and the presence of abnormalities of cerebrospinal fluid. It is the gold standard for neuroimaging in the emergent setting and for monitoring areas of hemorrhage and hydrocephalus in the first 1–4 weeks.

Magnetic Resonance Imaging

■ Magnetic resonance imaging (MRI) are 2-dimensional reconstructions of intracranial structures using variable movement and contents of hydrogen in tissues that are useful to detect very small masses, hemorrhage, and abnormalities of brain tissue. MR images can be manipulated via programming adjustments to detect specific abnormalities of white matter (diffusion tension imaging), brain edema and inflammation (FLAIR sequence), blood flow (magnetic resonance angiography), and other conditions. While it has limited utility in the emergent period, there is a suggestion that early evidence of diffuse axonal injury of the white matter may prognosticate for a poor functional outcome. MRIs may be used to assess patients who have persistent symptoms at the end of a period of expected recovery (eg, after 1–3 months in mild TBI, after 3–6 months in moderate TBI, after 6–12 months in severe TBI) to assess for the degree of brain damage.

Positive Emission Tomography, Single Photon Emission Computed Tomography, and Functional Magnetic Resonance Imaging

- These are the three most commonly used types of dynamic neuroimaging.
- Dynamic neuroimaging includes techniques that assess the metabolic (eg, oxygen utilization, glucose utilization) activity of the brain, such as with SPECT or PET scanning, or that uses standard structural imaging (ie, MRI) applied during the performance of standardized activities (eg, moving a finger, visualizing an image), such as with fMRI. The specific clinical applications of these newer techniques are still being elucidated.

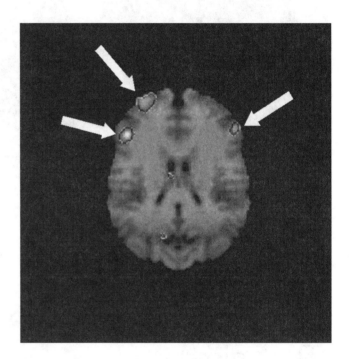

An example of O-15 positive emission tomography combined with an activation paradigm. The participant is being asked to recall a previously learned list of words while being scanned. Regions of increased blood flow (indicated by the arrows) within the frontal lobes are associated with increased cerebral activity known to mediate retrieval of newly learned information. (With permission from Zasler ND, Katz DI, Zafonte RD. *Brain Injury Medicine: Principles and Practice.* New York: Demos Medical Publishing; 2007.)

Diagnostic Tests: Swallowing

Modified Barium Swallow

- A modified barium swallow or videofluorography is the gold standard test for swallowing, performed with varying consistencies (eg, liquid, semisolid, solid) of barium and observed real-time with fluoroscopy. Delayed or absent swallowing reflex, aspiration, and oral phase dysfunction are the most common abnormalities found on videofluoroscopy. While small, there is radiation exposure with videofluorography.

Fiberoptic Endoscopic Evaluation of Swallowing

- Fiberoptic endoscopic evaluation of swallowing (FEES) is a real-time observation of swallowing. FEES has two main limitations: (a) cannot visualize oral and esophageal swallowing phases and (b) does not evaluate the initial elevation of the larynx or contraction of the pharynx during the pharyngeal phase. Limited viewing of actual swallow limits utility.

Diagnostic Tests: Vascular

Venous Duplex Ultrasonography

- Venous ultrasound is used to assess the patency of the venous system. It is primarily used to detect acute and chronic venous thrombosis. While highly useful in the lower leg/forearm and thigh/arm, it has limited sensitivity in the upper thigh/pelvis and shoulder.

Contrast Venography

- The "gold standard" technique to assess the patency of the venous system, it consists of contrast dye injected into the venous system and observed using fluoroscopy. It is limited by its cost, painfulness, and risk (1%–3%) of thrombosis.

D-dimer

- The D-dimer blood test is used to assess the amount of circulating thrombotic breakdown products (ie, D-dimer), as a screening tool for venous thrombosis. While easy to obtain and highly sensitive, it has limited specificity and little clinical utility.

Triple Phase Bone Scan

- A triple phase bone scan measures the ability of the body to absorb Technecium-99 over a 3-hour period and is used to determine signs of acute inflammation. The three phases, flow (immediate), perfusion (1–5 min) and reuptake (3 h) can be used to identify the acuity of inflammation, specifically in the diagnoses of joint infection and heterotopic ossification. The final phase is more commonly used to assess for stress fractures of bones.

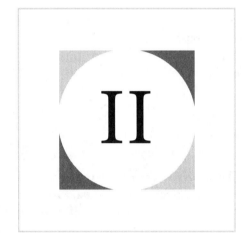

II Conditions

Agitation and Restless Behavior

Description
- Emotional state of excitement, restlessness, or excess psychomotor activity related to altered behavioral control from TBI.
- Level of behaviors range from poor impulse control to irritability to frank aggression
- Considered a stage of recovery in moderate to severe TBI (Ranchos Las Amigos level IV)
- In mild TBI, may present with initially subtle behavioral difficulties (poor frustration tolerance, decreased interpersonal skills, irritability)
- Occurs in approximately 11% to 50% of patients with moderate to severe TBI

Etiology
- May be seen in injuries affecting focal subcortical (limbic system) and cortical (temporal lobe) structures but is most commonly related to frontal lobe-mediated behavioral control issues
- Temporal lobe epilepsy may present with acute increase in agitated behavior.

Risk Factors
- Frontal lobe lesion
- Temporal lobe lesion
- Premorbid personality disorders
- Alcohol and substance abuse issues pre- and postinjury

Clinical Features
- Major morbidity of TBI
- Usually related to posttraumatic amnesia and thus seen more commonly in the acute phase after injury
- May see verbal and physical aggression directed toward self or others
- Interferes with daily functioning
- Typically short-lived in recovering moderate and severe TBI (2 weeks) but can persist
- Improvements in cognition (especially orientation) typically occur in concert with the start of agitation.

Diagnosis

Differential diagnosis
- Delirium
- Mania (± bipolar disease)
- Adverse reaction from medication
- Substance abuse
- Acute alcohol intoxication and/or withdrawal
- Benzodiazepine withdrawal
- Seizures
- Hyperthyroidism

History
- H/o substance abuse
- H/o acute alcohol abuse
- H/o personality disorder

Exam
- Evaluate for potential treatable sources of pain
- Assessment of cognitive (orientation) status

Testing
- Agitation Behavior Scale is a validated 14-point scale for objective measurement of agitation. Subscales can be used to assess for components of agitation: aggression, disinhibition/irritability, and emotional lability.

Pitfalls
- Behavior following TBI is often variable, so assessment should be done at multiple time points and by varied clinicians/observers.

Red Flags
- Acute worsening of agitation can be indicative of temporal lobe epilepsy, acute medication effect, new or worsened delirium, or substance use.

Treatment

Conservative
- One-to-one monitoring
- Physical restraints (including veiled beds)
- Behavioral management and modification techniques
- Environmental modification
- Medical management consists of reduction of pain, parenteral tubes, IV lines and eliminating other noxious stimuli that may be contributing to behavior.

Medical
- Minimize benzodiazepines and typical antipsychotics
- Anticonvulsants, neurostimulants, and beta blockers can be used concomitantly to lessen agitation.
- Manage sleep hygiene

Exercises
- None

Surgical
- None

Consults
- Psychiatry for complex diagnostic and medication management

Complications/side effects
- Prompt management of agitated behavior is important to maintain engagement of team and family in patient care.
- Neuroleptic malignant syndrome
  - Not dose- or exposure-dependent
- Neuroleptics may lead to akathisia.
  - Resembles agitation that may lead to escalation of neuroleptic dose

Prognosis
- Excellent during acute period and for rapid onset but poor after 8 weeks

Helpful Hints
- Episodes of acute agitated behavior, especially if accompanied with willful or inadvertent striking of another person, often severely disrupt the treatment team's ability to provide appropriate care. A focused team meeting to discuss the patient's status, the agitated episode, and a coordinated therapeutic approach is warranted.

Suggested Reading
Sandel M, Mysiw W. The agitated brain injured patient. Part 1: Definitions, differential diagnosis, and assessment. *Arch Phys Med Rehabil* 77(6):617–623.

Mysiw W, Sandel M. The agitated brain injured patient. Part 2: Pathophysiology and treatment. *Arch Phys Med Rehabil* 78(2):213–220.

Section II: Conditions

Akinetic Mutism

Description
- State of consciousness with preserved awareness, retention of ability to move and speak but failure to do so (immobile and mute, but eyes open; follows environment but does not respond to commands)
- Patients do not display emotions.

Etiology
- Usually due to frontal lobe injury
- May be iatrogenically induced by the bilateral anterior cingulate lesions occasionally used to manage severe psychosis
- Also can be due to bilateral subcortical paramedian diencephalic and midbrain lesions or bilateral globus pallidus lesions

Risk Factors
- Damage to prefrontal limbic structures

Clinical Features
- Patients display severe apathy

Diagnosis

Differential diagnosis
- Abulia: milder on spectrum of akinetic mutism with reduced impulse to act, slow responses (lack of initiative and spontaneity)
- Apathy: a dull emotional tone; patient able to verbalize this lack of interest
- Depression: as flat affect, apathy
- Catatonia: associated with immobility and mutism due to psychiatric disease
- Extrapyramidal muteness due to Parkinsonism
- Subclinical status epilepticus
- Locked-in state: inability to move or talk due to quadriparesis and bulbar paralysis, only vertical eye movements and eye blinking may be preserved
- Persistent vegetative state: the loss of cortical function, no purposeful movements, and unaware of environment but alertness / sleep–wake cycles retained
- Aphemia: cortical anarthria but preserved nonverbal and written behavior

History
- Prior history of neuroleptic use
- Prior history of Parkinson disease
- Prior history of depression

Exam
- Assessment of verbal and nonverbal communication skills
- Assessment of strength, tone, and coordination

Testing
- Electroencephalogram

Pitfalls
- Severely impaired patients may be mistaken for being comatose.

Red Flags
- Variable performance may suggest acute intracranial process or psychological overlay.

Treatment

Medical
- Neurostimulants may be helpful.
- Dopaminergic agents may be helpful.

Exercises
- None

Modalities
- None

Surgical
- None

Consults
- Neurology

Complications/side effects
- None

Prognosis
- Poor prognosis for full recovery

Helpful Hints
- Akinetic mutism is a function of motor/speech initiation and can often be overcome with automatic

activity (eg, patient will be able to answer cell phone), whereas locked-in-syndrome is due to true motor paralysis.

Suggested Reading

Marin RS, Wilkosz PA. Disorders of diminished motivation. *J Head Trauma Rehabil* 2005;20(4):377–388.

Aphasia, Expressive (Motor)

Description
- Nonfluent language impairment
- Also known as Broca's aphasia
- A transcortical motor aphasia is similar to a Broca's aphasia, except repetition is intact.
- Individuals with Broca's aphasia frequently speak short, meaningful phrases that are produced with great effort.

Etiology
- Lesions in left inferior frontal cortex
- Direct lesion to the left inferior frontal cortex (Brodmann area 44 and 45)

Risk Factors
- Dominant middle cerebral artery circulation disturbance

Clinical Features
- Effortful speech
- Restricted vocabulary
- Auditory comprehension usually intact
- Writing severely impaired
- Variable reading deficit
- Impaired repetition

Diagnosis

Differential diagnosis
- Wernicke aphasia (+fluency, −repetition, −comprehension)
- Global aphasia (−fluency, −repetition, −comprehension)
- Transcortical motor aphasia (−fluency, +repetition, −comprehension)
- Transcortical sensory aphasia (−fluency, +repetition, −comprehension)
- Anomic aphasia (+fluency, +repetition, +comprehension)—word finding difficulties
- Conduction aphasia (+fluency, − repetition, +comprehension)

History
- Prior language deficits
- Evaluation of baseline literacy, language, and educational limitations
- Baseline hearing deficits
- Acute or chronic tracheal or vocal cord dysfunction, eg, intubation trauma

Exam
- Assess fluency
- Assess repetition
- Assess for paraphrases—incorrect word or sound substitutions
- Assess for neologisms—made up words
- Assess comprehension of verbal orders
- Assess reading
- Assess writing

Testing
- Boston Diagnostic Aphasia Examination
- Western Aphasia Battery

Pitfalls
- Illiteracy
- New or preexisting hearing deficits

Red Flags
- A heightened level of anxiety in a patient with limited communication may be a sign of acute medical issues (eg, acute pain, myocardial infarction, pulmonary embolus).

Treatment

Medical
- Communication boards
- Case reports of the benefits of bromocriptine but not proven in randomized double blind placebo controlled trial

Exercises
- Melodic intonation therapy
- Constraint induced speech therapy = communication without gesturing or pointing

Modalities
- May be a role for assistive technology

Surgical
- None

Consults
- Speech language pathology

Prognosis
- Improvements in outcome associated with intensity of treatment

Helpful Hints
- Overlearned words (eg, expletives), phrases (eg, "how are you") and songs (eg, Happy Birthday) may be the first to return with severe aphasia.

Suggested Reading

Goodglass H, ed. *The Assessment of Aphasia and Related Disorders.* Philadelphia, PA: Lea & Febiger.

Levin HS, Grossman RG, Kelly PJ. Aphasic disorder in patients with closed head injury. *J Neurol Neurosurg Psychiatry* 1976;39:1062–1070.

Aphasia, Receptive (Sensory)

Description
- Disturbance in language that affects comprehension
- Also known as Wernicke's aphasia
- A transcortical sensory aphasia is similar to a Wernicke's aphasia, except repetition is intact.
- Wernicke's aphasia will result in poor auditory and reading comprehension, and fluent, but nonsensical, oral and written expression.
- Individuals with Wernicke's aphasia usually have great difficulty understanding the speech of both themselves and others and are therefore often unaware of their mistakes.

Etiology
- Damage to the left superior temporal region
- Occasionally due to inferior parietal cortex damage (Brodmann area 22)
- Ischemia of the inferior division of left MCA

Risk Factors
- None

Clinical Features
- Impaired auditory comprehension
- Fluent speech
- Normal prosody
  - May give the impression that patient is speaking foreign language if using neologisms
- Fair to good grammar
- Verbal paraphasic errors
- Occasionally logorrhea: continuous speech
- Pressured speech: rapid sentences
- Often unaware of own deficits
- Repetition deficit must be present for diagnosis of Wernicke aphasia.

Diagnosis

Differential diagnosis
- Broca aphasia (–fluency, –repetition, +comprehension)
- Global aphasia (–fluency, –repetition, –comprehension)
- Transcortical motor aphasia (–fluency, +repetition, –comprehension)
- Transcortical sensory aphasia (+fluency, +repetition, –comprehension)
- Anomic aphasia (+fluency, +repetition, +comprehension)—word finding difficulties
- Conduction aphasia (+fluency,–repetition, +comprehension)

History
- Prior language deficits
- Evaluation of baseline literacy, language, and educational limitation
- Baseline hearing deficits

Exam
- Assess fluency
- Assess repetition
- Assess for paraphrases—incorrect word or sound substitutions
- Assess for neologisms—made up words
- Assess comprehension of verbal orders
- Assess reading
- Assess writing

Testing
- Boston Diagnostic Aphasia Examination
- Western Aphasia Battery

Pitfalls
- Illiteracy
- New or preexisting hearing deficits
- Cognitive deficits will compound communication deficits.

Red Flags
- Fluctuating or worsening deficits may indicate active process (worsening edema, hydrocephalus, seizures) or acute intoxication (medication effect, alcohol).

Treatment

Medical
- None

Exercises
- Speech and language pathology

Modalities
- May be a role for assistive technology

Surgical
- None

Consults
- Speech and language pathology

Complications/side effects
- None

Prognosis
- Less improvement compared to Broca aphasia

Helpful Hints
- Individuals with cognitive deficits and receptive aphasia will demonstrate greater receptive language deficits.

Suggested Reading

Goodglass H, ed. *The Assessment of Aphasia and Related Disorders.* Philadelphia, PA: Lea & Febiger.

Levin HS, Grossman RG, Kelly PJ. Aphasic disorder in patients with closed head injury. *J Neurol Neurosurg Psychiatry* 1976;39:1062–1070.

Section II: Conditions

Attentional Deficits, Mild Traumatic Brain Injury

Description
- Attentional deficits include distractibility, slowed thinking, and difficulty concentrating
- Attentional deficits are a prominent characteristic of mild TBI.

Etiology
- Three main centers for attention:
  - Posterior attention network: the parietal cortex, pulvinar and reticular thalamic nucleus, and superior colliculus are involved in orientation of sensory stimuli in space.
  - Anterior attention network: The anterior cingulate gyrus and supplemental motor area focus on target stimuli and inhibit attention to irrelevant stimuli.
  - Vigilance network: The locus coeruleus and brainstem/lateral frontal cortex communications maintain alertness.

Risk Factors
- Prior history of attentional dysfunction
- Injuries to frontal lobes

Clinical Features
- Slowed reaction time but often still accurate in responses
- May see detectable occult impairments with more complex tasks, especially in setting of competing stimuli
- Tasks that are usually automatic (driving, reading) may now require effortful concentration.

Diagnosis

Differential diagnosis
- Depression
- Substance abuse
- Sleep deprivation
- Posttraumatic headache
- Attention deficit/hyperactivity disorder
- Special sensory deficits (hearing, vision)

History
- History of attention difficulties, including ADHD
- Centrally acting medications

Exam
- Forward and backward digit span
- Spelling forward and backward
- Immediate recall

Testing
- Paced Auditory Serial Addition Test—measures speed of information processing by requiring the individual to perform serial additions over four trials of increasing speeds
- Concentration-Endurance Test—measures focused attention via a cancellation task in which randomly interspersed targets need to be cancelled out of a row of characters
- Brief Test of Attention – tests for divided attention by having the individual listen to string of numbers and letters. In the first part, the individual counts number of letters and in the second part counts number of numbers.
- Conners' Continuous Performance Test—tests for sustained attention via a 20-minute computerized module
- Attention Rating Scale: self report measure of attention in TBI

Pitfalls
- Attentional deficits of mild TBI are more easily elicited with dual task demands than with individual tasks on neuropsychological testing.

Red Flags
- Variable or worsening deficits may be indicative of a new problem, as TBI is a static event that typically improves for 18 months after the initial period of injury.

Treatment

Medical

- Neurostimulants (methylphenidate, dextroamphetamine)
- Amantadine

Exercises/rehabilitation

- Attention process training via cognitive exercises based on neuropsychological theory (ie, Attention Process Training)
- Self management strategies and environmental modifications (pacing strategies, key ideas log via tape recorder or message pad, avoidance of noisy places, eliminating environmental distractions, setting up filing systems, "do not disturb" signs posted at work).
- Use of external aids that help individual track and maintain organization (written checklists, electronic organizers, voice activated message recorders, key finders, pill box reminders).
- Psychosocial support to lessen social factors exacerbating attentional deficits (supported listening, relaxation training)

Modalities

- Devices used to reduce distraction (eg, ruler below text to assist in reading)

Surgical

- None

Consults

- Neuropsychology

Complications/side effects

- None

Prognosis

- Vast majority of individuals with attentional deficits after TBI will demonstrate improvements for first 12–18 months.

Helpful Hints

- Tests requiring increased complexity may be needed to detect attentional deficits in mild TBI.
- Behavioral (stress syndromes, depression, anxiety), medication effects, and pain may worsen attentional deficits after TBI.

Suggested Reading

Stuss DT, Stethem LL, Hugenholtz H, Picton T, Pivik J, Richard MT. Reaction time after head injury: Fatigue, divided and focused attention, and consistency of performance. *J Neurol Neurosurg Psychiatry* 1989;52:742–748.

Section II: Conditions

Balance Deficits

Description
- Balance is the maintenance of bodily equilibrium or stability.
- Balance is achieved through the interaction and coordination of visual, vestibular, and somatosensory information; motor control (muscle strength and tone); and skeletal integrity (joint range of motion, boney stability).
- Vertigo is the illusion of movement.
- Dizziness may include lightheadedness, presyncope, being unsteady, loss of balance, or vertigo.
- Presyncope is most often described as lightheaded or feeling faint. Presyncope, or lightheadedness, does not result from primary central nervous system pathology.

Etiology
- Increased intracranial pressure with intracranial or brainstem compression, or midline shift
- Cerebellar injury
- Ocular/optic tract injury
- Auditory or vestibular injury

Risk Factors
- Lower Glasgow Coma Score, acute craniotomy, longer length of coma, longer posttraumatic amnesia, and longer acute care length of stay are associated with impaired sitting balance and standing balance scores at admission to inpatient rehabilitation.
- Initial abnormalities in pupillary response are associated with impairments in sitting balance.
- Midline shift or brainstem compression on CT scan is associated with standing balance impairment on admission to inpatient rehabilitation.

Clinical Features
- Impairment in sitting balance can affect feeding, bathing, grooming, wheelchair mobility, and dressing.
- The more impaired the sitting balance, the more likely the need for assistance with activities of daily living (ADLs).
- After age, the most powerful predictor of discharge total functional independence measure (FIM) score is the degree of sitting balance impairment.
- Standing balance will be affected before sitting balance.

Diagnosis

Differential diagnosis
- Benign paroxysmal positional vertigo
- Inner ear (labyrinthine) concussion with otolith dislodgement
  - Labyrinthitis
  - Vertebrobasiliar artery insufficiency
  - Orthostatic hypotension
  - Peripheral neuropathy
- Posterior column (spinal cord) damage
- Hypoglycemia
- Migrainous aura
- Central acting medications
- Alcohol intoxication

History
- Identify if precise feelings of instability are present (ie, vertigo vs presyncope) or if patient just has inability to balance.
- Identify prior balance or coordination deficits.

Exam
- Perform complete cranial nerve, motor, sensory, tone, and deep tendon reflex examination
- Examine for dysdiadochokinesia (inability to perform rapid alternating movements)
- Examine for visual acuity and nystagmus
- Examine finger-to-nose and heel-to-shin testing
- Examine sitting and standing balance
- Assess gait with eyes open and closed

Testing
- Medical evaluation for hypoglycemia, hypoxia, and hypotension
- Assess for orthostatic hypotension (systolic blood pressure decrease of at least 20 mm Hg or a diastolic blood pressure decrease of at least 10 mm Hg within 3 minutes of standing)
- Caloric testing (measure of pupillary findings and subjective report of vertigo in response to cold water injected into the ear canals), if vertigo suspected

- Electronystagmography (electrophysiologic measure of pupillary response to vertical and horizontal visual stimuli), if nystagmus present
- Dix-Hallpike maneuver (assessment of the individual's response to rapid movement from sitting to lying with head rotated) to assess for benign paroxysmal positional vertigo
- Berg Balance Score (BBS): 14-item scale used to assess balance; however, does not assess gait
- Timed Get Up and Go test (the time required to rise from sitting, ambulate a distance, and return to the original seated position) assesses sit to stand, standing balance, gait, and turning balance.
- Computerized posturography (a measure of dynamic standing activities on a force plate) provides objective assessment of labyrinthian, visual, and proprioceptive pathways of balance.

Pitfalls
- Formal documentation of balance (eg, using the BBS) is not typically performed.

Red Flags
- Signs of hydrocephalus (worsened cognitive deficits, incontinence)
- Perilymphatic fistula (caused by disruption of the oval window) will cause sudden or progressive fluctuating sensorineural hearing loss and vertigo.

Treatment

Medical
- No proven medication benefit

Exercises
- Core strengthening
- Postural exercises focused on progressive head and trunk movements in space.
- Use of visual (mirror), auditory (bells), and kinesthetic (weights) cues during activity
- Aquatic-based rehabilitation activities
- Assistive devices
- Treadmill-assisted or Lokomat (robotic) gait therapy may be used.

Modalities
- None

Surgical
- None

Consults
- Otolaryngology

Complications/side effects
- Falls

Prognosis
- Rehabilitation admission standing balance correlates with ambulation at discharge.
- Rehabilitation sitting and standing balance correlates with the need for ADL assistance at rehabilitation discharge and at 1 year.
- Unsupported sitting balance correlates with length of stay.

Helpful Hints
- Acute use of central acting medications for imbalance (meclizine, dimenhydrinate, benozodiazepines) is contraindicated, as they may interfere with the brain's ability to recalibrate; however they may play a use in those with chronic difficulties.

Suggested Reading
Basford JR, Chou L-S, Kaufman KR, Brey RH, Walker A, Malec JF, Moessner AM, Brown AW. An assessment of gait and balance deficits after traumatic brain injury. *Arch Phys Med Rehabil* 2003;84:343–349.

Pickett TC, Radfar-Baublitz LS, McDonald SD, Walker WC, Cifu DX. Objectively assessing balance deficits after TBI: Role of computerized posturography. *J Rehab Res Dev* 2007;44(7):983–990.

Section II: Conditions

Bladder Issues

Description
- The most common bladder abnormality after brain injury is incontinence, although this is related to cognitive awareness (ie, frontal lobe control) in >98% of individuals. This is an unusual long-term sequela.

Etiology
- Volitional control of bladder function is controlled by the frontal lobes; incontinence may be seen when either direct or indirect (ie, disconnection between the frontal lobe and other structures) injury occurs.
- Injuries affecting the brainstem could also impact the upper cervical spinal cord and cause an upper motor neuron (spastic) bladder disorder.

Risk Factors
- Frontal lobe injury
- Severe brain injury
- Brainstem injury
- Preinjury urinary incontinence
- Prostatic hypertrophy with outflow obstruction

Clinical Features
- When caused by unawareness with poor volitional control, there will most commonly be bladder accidents when the bladder is filled (approximately 250 cc).
- As cognition improves, increasing control of urinary continence is seen.
- A spastic bladder will often result in significant urinary retention due to a spastic external sphincter. Without intervention, the bladder will only empty at large volumes (> 500 cc) related to overflow incontinence and there will be an elevated risk of hydronephrosis.

Diagnosis

Differential diagnosis
- Bladder accidents related to decreased mobility or communication skills
- Occult spinal cord injury
- Diabetic autonomic neuropathy
- Retention related to medications or immobility
- Retention or incontinence related to outflow obstruction or infectious cause
- Behavioral issues
- Occult injury to external sphincter

History
- Prior bladder accidents
- Prior frequency of voiding
- Prior history of urinary retention

Exam
- Perform complete cognitive examination
- Assess communication skills
- Assess mobility skills, including balance
- Examine the abdomen and pelvis, evaluating tenderness, bladder fullness, external genitalia
- Assess perineal and perianal sensation
- Perform anorectal examination, assessing for evidence of anal trauma or injury, integrity of anal sphincter, presence of anal wink and bulbocavernosum reflexes, pain, and status of rectal vault (presence of stool or mass, stool guaiac)

Testing
- Urinalysis with culture and sensitivity
- Urodynamics

Pitfalls
- Multiple hospital-related factors may affect bladder habits and continence (infection, diet and hydration, medications, activity, humility).
- Multiple TBI factors may affect bladder continence (cognition, behavior, mobility, communication).

Red Flags
- Change in quality (color, odor, clarity) or quantity of urine
- Evidence of infection (fever, chills, elevated white blood cell count)
- Pain with voiding

Treatment

Medical
- Limited role for bladder-specific medications acutely after TBI; incontinence will improve with cognition improvements.
- Probable negative effect of anticholinergic bladder agents (oxybutynin, tamsulosin) on cognition limits usage of these bladder relaxation agents.

- Medications to improve prostatic hypertrophy-related outflow obstruction may be helpful in males with urinary retention after TBI (often exacerbated by the inability to stand during voiding).
- Medications (hormones) to improve urethral atrophy in postmenopausal women may improve urinary incontinence.
- Little role for agents that stimulate urinary contraction (bethanocol)
- Urinary tract infections should be appropriately treated.

Exercises/rehabilitation

- Timed voiding (every 2–4 hours) may assist with behavioral training in cognitively unaware patients.
- No role for indwelling foley catheter, except for acute management of urinary retention or if fluid output must be closely monitored. High risk for behavioral worsening with indwelling catheter.
- A condom catheter may be appropriate if male patient cannot be kept dry between scheduled voids; however, skin must be monitored closely for breakdown.
- Diapers should be avoided if possible (may reinforce incontinent behavior, elevate risk for skin irritation)
- For spastic bladder, a scheduled program of intermittent catheterization is necessary, maintaining volumes 200–500 cc.

Modalities

- N/A

Surgical

- N/A

Consults

- N/A

Complications/side effects

- Elevated risk of skin irritation and breakdown with incontinence. Meticulous perineal care, close monitoring, and the use of protective skin products are required.
- Elevated risk of recurrent urinary tract infection and hydronephrosis with spastic bladder

Prognosis

- It is rare to see long-term bladder incontinence after TBI.

Helpful Hints

- New urinary tract infection, medication with cognitive side effects, or a change in fluid intake (PO, IV) are common sources for worsening urinary continence.

Suggested Reading

Chua K, Chuo A, Kong KH. Urinary incontinence after traumatic brain injury: Incidence, outcomes and correlates. *Brain Inj* 2003;17(6):469–478.

Section II: Conditions

Bowel Issues

Description
- The most common bowel abnormality after brain injury is incontinence, although this is related to cognitive awareness (ie, frontal lobe control) in >98% of individuals. This is an unusual long-term sequela.

Etiology
- Volitional control of bowel function is controlled by the frontal lobe; incontinence may be seen when either direct or indirect (ie, disconnection between the frontal lobe and other structures) injury occurs.
- Injuries affecting the brainstem can impact the upper cervical spinal cord and cause an upper motor neuron (spastic) bowel disorder.

Risk Factors
- Frontal lobe injury
- Severe brain injury
- Brainstem injury

Clinical Features
- When caused by unawareness with poor volitional control, there will most commonly be bowel accidents when the colonic vault is overfilled. Early in the course of injury, stool will be well formed and bowel movements occur regularly (ie, after meals); however, if incontinence persists, it is common for the vault to release small amounts of stool throughout the day.
- As cognition improves, increasing control of bowel movements is seen.
- A spastic bowel will often result in significant obstipation due to a spastic external sphincter. Without intervention, stooling will be infrequent and copious.

Diagnosis

Differential diagnosis
- Bowel accidents related to decreased mobility or communication skills
- Occult spinal cord injury
- Diabetic autonomic neuropathy
- Obstipation related to medications or immobility
- Diarrhea related to obstipation, malabsorption, or infectious cause
- Behavioral issues
- Occult injury to external sphincter

History
- Prior bowel accidents
- Prior schedule of bowel movements
- Prior constipation or diarrhea
- Prior use/abuse of bowel medications and agents

Exam
- Perform complete cognitive examination
- Assess communication skills
- Assess mobility skills, including balance
- Examine the abdomen, evaluating tenderness, bowel sounds, masses
- Assess perineal and perianal sensation
- Perform anorectal examination, assessing for evidence of anal trauma or injury, integrity of anal sphincter, presence of anal wink and bulbocavernosum reflexes, pain, and status of rectal vault (presence of stool or mass, stool guaiac)

Testing
- Stool evaluation for infection (clostridium difficile enteritis)
- Bowel manometry

Pitfalls
- Multiple hospital-related factors may affect bowel habits and continence (infection, diet and hydration, medications, activity, antibiotic usage, humility).
- Multiple TBI factors may affect bowel continence (cognition, behavior, mobility, communication).

Red Flags
- Worsening continence is not typical in recovering TBI.
- Diarrhea is not typical in TBI, and therefore other sources should be sought.

Treatment

Medical
- Stool softeners for physically limited patients
- No bowel-specific medications for continence
- Spastic bowel typically requires a scheduled bowel program every 1–2 days.

Exercises/rehabilitation

- Placing the patient on the toilet after meals (or tube feeds) on a regular basis may assist in behavioral training.
- Diapers should be avoided if possible (may reinforce incontinent behavior, elevate risk for skin irritation).

Modalities

- N/A

Surgical

- N/A

Consults

- GI service for persistent diarrhea.

Complications/side effects

- Dehydration and/or electrolyte abnormalities are often seen with diarrhea.
- Constipation often results in abdominal discomfort and poor appetite, and while rare, constipation may lead to bowel obstruction or rupture.

- Elevated risk of skin irritation and breakdown with incontinence. Meticulous perineal care, close monitoring, and the use of protective skin products are required.

Prognosis

- It is rare to see long-term bowel incontinence after TBI.

Helpful Hints

- Tube feedings are a common source of diarrhea, especially when dosing or type changes.

Suggested Reading

Foxx-Orenstein A, Kolakowsky-Hayner S, Marwitz JH, et al. Incidence, risk factors, and outcomes of fecal incontinence after acute brain injury: Findings from the Traumatic Brain Injury Model Systems national database. *Arch Phys Med Rehabil* 2003;84:231–237.

Central Dysautonomia

Description
- Altered autonomic activity seen after TBI resulting in hypertension, fever, tachycardia, tachypnea, pupillary dilation, and extensor posturing.
- The term paroxysmal autonomic instability with dystonia (PAID) is also used.

Etiology
- Dysregulation of the autonomic system due to brainstem injury from trauma, bleeding, infection, or pressure
- Cortical areas that influence the activity of the hypothalamus include the orbitofrontal, anterior temporal, and insular regions. Subcortical areas that influence the hypothalamus include the amygdala (particularly the central nucleus), the periaqueductal gray matter, the nucleus of the tractus solitarius, the cerebellar uvula, and the cerebellar vermis. Damage to these areas releases control of vegetative functions and results in dysregulation of overall autonomic balance.
- Reported in up to 15% to 33% of individuals in coma or vegetative states

Risk Factors
- Severe brain injury
- Hydrocephalus
- Central nervous system infection

Clinical Features
- Clinical manifestations of dysautonomia consist of a temperature of ≥ 38.5°C, hypertension, a pulse rate of at least 130 beats per minute, a respiratory rate of at least 140 breaths per minute, intermittent agitation, and diaphoresis; these are accompanied by dystonia (rigidity or decerebrate posturing for a duration of at least one cycle per day for at least 3 days).
- Other issues that can occur because of autonomic dysregulation are electrocardiographic alterations, arrhythmias, increased intracranial pressure (ICP), hypohidrosis, subnormal temperature in flaccid limbs, and neurogenic lung disease.
- Usually episodic, PAID first appears in the intensive care setting but may persist into the rehabilitation

phase for weeks to months after injury in individuals who remain in a low-response state.

Diagnosis

Differential diagnosis
- Essential hypertension
- Hydrocephalus
- Sepsis
- Neuroleptic malignant syndrome
- Serotonin syndrome
- Malignant hyperthermia
- Thyroid storm
- Deep venous thrombosis and/or pulmonary emblous

History
- H/o dysautonomia
- H/o neuroleptic malignant syndrome
- H/o serotonin syndrome
- H/o malignant hyperthermia

Exam
- Standard general physical examination
- Standard TBI examination
- Neurologic examination

Testing
- Neuroimaging to rule out active processes (infection, bleeding, hydrocephalus)
- Chest X-ray to rule out acute process (pneumonia, pulmonary embolus, atelectasis, preexisting pulmonary disease)
- Doppler ultrasonography to rule out deep venous thrombosis
- EKG to rule out myocardial infarction or underlying cause for tachycardia
- Complete blood count (CBC) to assess for infection
- Blood cultures to assess for infection
- Sputum cultures to assess for infection
- Urine cultures and urinalysis to assess for infection
- Sputum gram stain to assess for infection
- Thyroid panel to assess for hyperthyroidosis
- Random chemistry panel to assess for sodium imbalance
- Plasma creatine kinase and troponin levels to rule out cardiac injury

Pitfalls

- Central dysautonomia is a diagnosis of exclusion; therefore more common causes of elevated temperature, blood pressure, respiratory rate and pulse should be investigated.

Red Flags

- Elevated white blood cell counts are consistent with infection, not PAID.
- Persistently abnormal vital signs are not typical of PAID.

Treatment

Medical

- Beta blockers and alpha adrenergic blockers are useful for hypertension.
- Bromocriptine has been used to help combat the hyperthermia and diaphoresis.
- Dantrolene has been a useful treatment for extensor posturing.
- Morphine and naltrexone have been used to manage central dysautonomia.
- Gabapentin may be effective in controlling the autonomic symptoms and the dystonic posturing.

Exercises/rehabilitation

- Limited participation in therapy is tolerated

Modalities

- N/A

Surgical

- N/A

Consults

- Infectious disease
- Neurosurgery

Complications/side effects

- Blood pressure and pulse spikes may result in stroke, myocardial infarction, and death.

Prognosis

- While often self-limited in the first several weeks, the presence of central dysautonomia is associated with a poor functional outcome after TBI.

Helpful Hints

- Eliminate any nonessential medications when assessing a patient with possible central dysautonomia.
- Completing a comprehensive evaluation in the second week of symptoms of central dysautonomia is recommended to allow for natural recovery while also reducing the risk of missing other diagnoses.

Suggested Reading

Baguleya IJ, Nicholls JL, Felmingham KL, Crooks J, Gurka JA, Wade LD. Dysautonomia after traumatic brain injury: A forgotten syndrome? *J Neurol Neurosurg Psychiatry* 1999;67:39–43.

Section II: Conditions

Cognitive Deficits of Traumatic Brain Injury

Description
- Cognitive deficits include impairment in attention, learning, memory, and executive functioning.
- Executive functioning refers to cognitive control or cognitive processes that guide behavior.
- Memory impairments include deficits in encoding, consolidation, and retrieval.

Etiology
- Primarily cortical lesions

Risk Factors
- Diffuse axonal injury
- Alcohol use pre- and peri-injury
- Hippocampus injury
- Prefrontal cortex injury
- Prior head trauma

Clinical Features
- Memory deficits are most profound initially after injury (posttraumatic amnesia).
- TBI affects episodic memory (recollection of personal events) more than procedural memory (occurring outside of conscious awareness).
- TBI often affects prospective memory or the ability to remember an individual's future intentions (forgetting appointments, forgetting to pay bills).
- May see deficit of metamemory, or self-awareness, of memory deficits.
- In mild TBI, unlike moderate to severe TBI, there may be spontaneous recovery of cognitive function.
- May see anosognosia (lack of acknowledgment of neurologic deficit)
- May see confabulations in the setting of significant memory loss

Diagnosis
Differential diagnosis
- Premorbid cognitive deficits (learning disabilities, ADHD)
- Posttraumatic amnesia
- Sleep deprivation
- Depression

History
- Assess for complicating factors including pain, sleep disturbances, depression, and stress

Exam
- Testing of cognitive skills

Testing
- Neuropsychological assessment
  - Standardized cognitive and behavioral evaluation using validated and normed testing performed in a formal environment
  - Specifically designed tasks used to measure a psychological function known to be linked to a particular brain structure or pathway
- Galveston Orientation and Amnesia Test

Pitfalls
- Neurolinguistic and language deficits may mimic cognitive deficits.
- Depression may mimic cognitive deficits (pseudodementia cerebri).

Red Flags
- Cognitive, balance, and continence deficits may be signs of hydrocephalus.

Treatment
Medical
- Limited evidence that medications have an impact on cognition,; however, the following classes may be considered:
  - Acetylcholinesterase inhibitors (donepezil)
  - Neurostimulants (methylphenidate)
  - SSRI (fluoxetine)
  - Dopaminergic agents (amantadine)

Exercises
- Neurocognitive rehabilitation

Modalities
- Personal digital assistant and programmed pagers can provide structured cueing
- Use of external aids that help individual track and maintain organization (written checklists, electronic

organizers, voice activated message recorders, key finders, pill box reminders).

Surgical
■ None

Consults
■ Neuropsychology

Complications/side effects
■ None

Prognosis
■ Anosognosia is associated with poorer outcome and more limited ability to participate in the rehabilitation progress.

Helpful Hints
■ Cognitive deficits typically contribute more to disability than do physical impairments.

■ Mild cognitive deficits may only be elucidated during dual task conditions.
■ Tests requiring increased complexity may be needed to detect cognitive deficits in mild TBI.
■ Behavioral (stress syndromes, depression, anxiety), medication effects, and pain may worsen cognitive deficits after TBI.

Suggested Reading

Arciniegas D, Adler L, Topkoff J, Cawthra E, Filley CM, Reite M. Attention and memory dysfunction after traumatic brain injury: Cholinergic mechanisms, sensory gating, and a hypothesis for further investigation. *Brain Inj* 1999;13:1–13.

McDowell S, Whyte J, D'Esposito M. Working memory impairments in traumatic brain injury: Evidence from a dual-task paradigm. *Neuropsychologia* 1997;35(10):1341–1353.

Combat-Related Traumatic Brain Injury

Description

- With the global war on terror (GWOT), marked increase in blast-related injuries (sources of blasts include mines, improvised explosive devices [IEDs], grenades, aerial bombs, mortar shells)
- In all, 60% of blast-related injuries seen at military trauma centers have TBI, with vast majority being mild TBIs.
- Higher rates of survival (>95% of all injuries) seen in twenty-first century warfare due to improvements in body armor and acute trauma care
- Unclear what percentage of brain injury is due to primary pressure gradient effects of blast wave versus secondary or tertiary effects of blast

Etiology

- Four components of a blast injury:
  - Primary: due to shock wave passing through body, unclear effect on brain; common cause of perforated tympanic membrane
  - Secondary: due to bomb fragments or other objects being propelled through the body (ie, penetrating brain injury)
  - Tertiary: due to blast wind effect on the victim; may cause amputation, bony fractures, falls with TBI (ie, acceleration-deceleration or blunt trauma-related TBI)
  - Quaternary: burns, respiratory injuries, and crushing injuries (ie, hypoxic or ischemic brain injury)

Risk Factors

- Proximity to blast epicenter increases injury and severity of TBI.

Clinical Features

- Blast injuries are usually polytraumatic, involving more than one body system.
- May see comorbid posttraumatic stress disorder (PTSD) related to blast exposure

Diagnosis

Differential diagnosis

- Combat-related stress disorders
- Psychosocial overlay related to malingering, secondary gain (benefits, service connectiveness)
- Combat-related mild TBI often accompanied by post-traumatic stress disorder
- Alcohol/drug usage

History

- Standard TBI history
- Prior exposures to blast
- Military branch, rank, and responsibilities
- Prior TBI

Exam

- Standard TBI exam

Testing

- Consider neuroimaging and/or neuropsychology testing for symptoms that are not consistent with injury or injury severity

Pitfalls

- Many service members are trained to downplay symptoms or may not acknowledge them to maintain military readiness.
- Acuteness of battlefield and of concomitant polytraumatic injuries often prevents a detailed assessment of neurologic status (especially in mild TBI).

Red Flags

- Multiple blast exposure or reports of TBI

Treatment

- Rehabilitation environments with military-specific personnel and tasks that address issues relevant to service members allow for optimal care.

Medical

- Standard treatments for TBI

Exercises
- Standard treatments for TBI

Modalities
- None

Surgical
- None

Consults
- Mental health professionals for stress and anxiety issues

Complications/side effects
- Combat-related moderate or severe TBI may have made multi-system (polytrauma) complications than non-combat injuries

Prognosis
- Blasts produce unique injuries but are not an independent predictor of functional outcome.

Helpful Hints
- Use standard TBI assessment and management strategies initially, regardless of concomitant conditions (eg, PTSD, pain syndromes).

Suggested Reading
Sayer NA, Cifu DX, McNamee S, et al. Rehabilitation needs of combat-injured service members admitted to the VA poly-trauma rehabilitation centers: The role of PM&R in the care of wounded warriors. *PM&R* 2009;1(1):23–28.

Concussion: Cumulative Mild Traumatic Brain Injury

Description
- Multiple concussions (three or more) over the course of lifetime, with potential for traumatic encephalopathy with progressive functional difficulties and early death

Etiology
- Stretching of axons that leads to structural damage and metabolic dysfunction

Risk Factors
- Contact sports
  - Boxing or ultimate fighting
  - Heading soccer balls
  - In football: ball return carriers, quarterbacks, tight ends, and linebackers
- Combat injuries with multiple blast exposures

Clinical Features
- Symptoms range from asymptomatic to mild cognitive and memory impairments to severe chronic encephalopathy.
- "Punch drunk syndrome" or "dementia pugilistica"—extrapyramidal and cerebellar dysfunction signs in addition to cognitive behavioral abnormalities seen in boxers during or after their fighting career.
- May see progressive cognitive and behavioral dysfunction (dementia)
- Anxiety is seen as a more troublesome symptom as concussions accumulate
- Cognitive deficits appear earlier than would commonly be associated with vascular or Alzheimer dementia.

Diagnosis

Differential diagnosis
- Other causes of progressive dementia

- Secondary insult to the brain (eg, vascular infarct) may contribute to deficits

History
- History of concussion

Exam
- Full neurologic exam

Testing
- Neuropsychological testing may help to define nature of preexisting and new deficits.
- Neuroimaging to rule out other non-TBI sources of deficits

Pitfalls
- Normal pressure hydrocephalus is a progressive dementing process from TBI that may respond to treatment (shunting).

Red Flags
- Extrapyramidal or cerebellar signs

Treatment

Medical
- Manage secondary risk factors for brain insult

Exercises
- None

Modalities
- Unclear role for cognitive therapy, but reasonable to deliver services

Surgical
- None

Consults
- Neuropsychology

Complications/side effects
- See Combat-Related Traumatic Brain Injury (page 46)

Prognosis

- Typically excellent recovery after initial injury but declines with subsequent injury

Helpful Hints

- Increased risk of depression
- Increased risk of postconcussive syndrome
- A player who receives three concussions in one season should be removed from play for the rest of the season.

Suggested Reading

Repetitive Head Injury Syndrome. Available at: http://emedicine. medscape.com/article/92189-overview.

Slemmer JE, Matser EJT, De Zeeuw CI, Weber JT. Repeated mild injury causes cumulative damage to hippocampal cells. *Brain* 2002;125(12):2699–2709.

Concussion: Mild Traumatic Brain Injury

Description
- Brief (< 30 minutes) alteration in consciousness after trauma to head, typically associated with transient neurologic sequelae and period of retrograde or anterograde memory loss

Etiology
- Usually the result of rapid acceleration/deceleration of head with transient disruption of axonal activity
- Primarily reversible neurometabolic pathophysiology
- Usually not associated with macroscopic changes on CT scan; however, diffuse axonal injury (white matter tract hemorrhage) is the most common finding
- Magnetic resonance imaging (MRI) is the best modality to see acute abnormalities

Risk Factors
- History of concussion
- Rapid acceleration-deceleration of head as seen with motor vehicle collisions or with blunt trauma to head in sports

Clinical Features
- Alteration or loss of consciousness of less than 30 minutes
- Transient confusion
- Memory dysfunction around the time of injury
- Transient signs of neurologic/neuropsychological dysfunction (seizures, irritability, lethargy, vomiting, headaches, dizziness, fatigue)

Diagnosis

Differential diagnosis
- Delirium related to alcohol or drug intoxication
- Acute stress disorder (first 3 months)
- Anxiety disorder
- Cognitive dysfunction related to pain, medication, or sleep deprivation
- Depression

History
- Identify specifics of injury and events/status surrounding time of injury
- If possible, verify injury specifics via emergency department and medical records, EMS run sheets, and witnesses.
- Prior concussion
- Preinjury drug or alcohol usage
- Use of helmet (sports)
- Use of vehicle restraints
- Airbag deployment

Exam
- Mental status assessment
- Full neurologic exam
- Depression screen

Testing
- CT scanning is (by definition) normal, except in the case of "complicated mild TBI" where small amounts of subarachnoid hemorrhage may be seen.
- Neuropsychological assessment of general intellectual ability, perception, judgment, verbal, and constructive and executive functions
- Balance testing
- Advanced neuroimaging (MRI) if history, exam, initial testing, and symptoms are not congruous (see Assessment Scales: Concussion Grading)

Pitfalls
- Events at time of injury must be carefully reviewed as close to injury as is possible to optimize diagnosis.
- Acute stress conditions may mimic mild TBI, except that a clear alteration or loss of consciousness is absent.

Red Flags
- No evidence for increased late seizure rate with concussion; consider non-TBI–related causes if there are seizures.
- New onset stuttering is nonphysiologic and a common sign of psychologic overlay.

Treatment

Medical

- Compensatory strategies for memory deficits (daily planners and calendars)
- Environmental modifications to minimize distraction
- Pragmatic approach to symptoms includes
  - Avoiding invalidating injury or symptoms
  - Promoting functional competence of individual
  - Promoting rapid return to activity
  - Vocational training

Exercises

- Symptoms specific interventions

Modalities

- None

Surgical

- None

Consults

- None

Complications/side effects

- See Concussion: Postconcussive Symptoms/Syndrome (page 52)

Prognosis

- In all, 15% to 30% of individuals will have persistent symptoms at 1 to 3 months, 3% at 1 year
- Have higher return-to-work rates than moderate or severe brain injury
- No clear association between mild TBI and risk for Alzheimer dementia, although there may be a subgroup at higher risk (Apo-E4)

Helpful Hints

- Cognitive symptoms can occur without loss of consciousness.
- Loss of consciousness cannot occur without cognitive symptoms.

Suggested Reading

McCrea M, Guskiewicz KM, Marshall SE. Acute effects and recovery time following concussion in collegiate football players: The NCAA Concussion Study. *JAMA* 2003;290:2556–2563.

Concussion: Postconcussive Symptoms/Syndrome (PCS)

Description

- Set of physical, cognitive, emotional, and behavioral symptoms that a person may experience 1- to 3 months after injury
- Usually associated with a mild TBI but can be seen after moderate-severe TBI
- Most common symptom is headache
- Patient must have persistence of three or more of the following symptoms: headaches, dizziness, fatigue, irritability, sleep problems, concentration problems, memory problems, and problems tolerating stress/alcohol/emotions.

Etiology

- Associated with TBI, but unclear causes

Risk Factors

- Most common with mTBI vs moderate or severe TBI
- Preexisting psychological disorders
- Expectations of disability
- Older age
- Low socioeconomic status
- Prior m TBI
- Recurrent TBI before symptoms of first have resolved
- Female gender
- History of alcohol abuse
- Traumatic memories of the event

Clinical Features

- While postconcussive symptoms are common after TBI, persistent symptoms and three or more symptoms are not.
- Research demonstrates that neurophysiologic abnormalities are worse in first 48 hours and rapidly return to normal baseline by 2 weeks postinjury.
- Symptoms are predominately physical in nature at onset of PCS but later progress to a more psychological presentation.
- Physical symptoms include headache, dizziness, fatigue, noise sensitivity, nausea, vomiting, light sensitivity, decreased sense of taste/smell, blurred vision, diplopia, tinnitus, and hearing loss and are typically present within the first 48 hours.

- Cognitive symptoms include memory deficits (especially short-term memory), difficulty concentrating, personality changes, and slowed information processing and are typically noticed within the first 2 weeks postinjury.
- Behavioral symptoms include irritability, poor judgment, restlessness, agitation, decreased libido, and impaired social interaction and may not be noticed for 4 weeks postinjury.
- Emotional symptoms include depression, anxiety, and lability.

Diagnosis

Differential diagnosis

- Malingering or symptom magnification (especially in cases of litigation)
- Posttraumatic stress disorder
- Major depressive disorder
- Fibromyalgia
- Vertebral artery dissection
- Hypopituitism
- Sleep deprivation

History

- Rivermead Postconcussive Symptoms Questionnaire—assesses 16 symptoms commonly found in PCS.
- Neurobehavioral Symptom Inventory—assesses 22 symptoms commonly found in PCS.
- Patient must have three of the following eight symptom-cluster within 4 weeks of injury (headaches, dizziness, fatigue, irritability, sleep problems, concentration problems, memory problems, problems tolerating stress/alcohol/emotions)

Exam

- Complete TBI physical examination

Testing

- Consider MRI scan in significantly symptomatic patients.
- Functional neuroimaging may detect impairments; however, this is rarely necessary.
- Neuropsychological testing to qualify and quantify cognitive and behavioral deficits and assist in defining psychological overlay

Pitfalls

■ Stress disorders, pain, depression, medication effects, and sleep deprivation can present with signs and symptoms that are similar to PCS.

Red Flags

■ New onset stuttering after TBI is nonphysiologic and an indicator of psychological overlay
■ Long-term memory deficits are not typical of PCS or mild TBI, and other causes should be evaluated.
■ Worsening symptoms are not typical for PCS or mild TBI, and other causes should be evaluated.

Treatment

Medical

■ See symptoms-specific chapters of this book.
■ Education of patient regarding common symptoms and excellent prognosis is major acute treatment.

Exercises

■ Rapid return to physical activity and work within limits of symptoms is therapeutic.
■ Restriction of all contact activities/sports until symptoms fully resolved
■ Activity limitations are required to avoid repeat TBI.

Modalities

■ None

Surgical

■ None

Consults

■ Neuropsychology

Complications/side effects

■ Persistent symptoms may be seen in 3–15% of injuries after 1 year.
■ Only symptoms present during acute (4 week) phase should be considered as related to TBI.

Prognosis

■ Cognitive symptoms tend to improve the fastest.
■ Excellent prognosis for functional recovery
■ In all, 15%–30% of mTBI will have PCS at 1–3 months and 3% at 1 year.
■ Poor prognosis with depression, chronic pain, post-traumatic stress disorder, substance abuse, ongoing litigation

Helpful Hints

■ Most clinicians have a poor understanding of mTBI and PCS.

Suggested Reading

Iverson GL. Outcome from mild traumatic brain injury. *Curr Opin Psychiatry* 2005;18:301–317.

Section II: Conditions

Concussion: Second Impact Syndrome

Description
- Rapid development of brain edema and herniation as a consequence of a second brain injury
- The second impact (brain injury) occurs prior to resolution of the first impact symptoms
- Extremely rare event

Etiology
- Loss of autoregulation of brain-blood supply leads to increased intracranial pressure and subsequent herniation of the temporal lobe or the cerebellar tonsils.

Risk Factors
- Residual symptoms from first brain injury including changes in visual, motor, and sensory processing in addition to memory or cognitive dysfunction

Clinical Features
- Second trauma may be minor, and athlete may not lose consciousness; seconds to minutes after second impact, the athlete collapses to the ground; rapidly dilated pupils, loss of eye movement, and respiratory failure ensues
- 50% mortality rate
- 100% morbidity rate

Diagnosis

Differential diagnosis
- Epidural hematoma
  - Frequently associated with fracture of temporal bone and subsequent tear of middle meningeal artery
  - See symptoms in 1– to 2 hours after impact.
  - Athlete may have lucid interval.
- Postictal paralysis (Todd palsy)
- Hypokalemic periodic paralysis
- Hyperkalemic periodic paralysis
- Pontine hemorrhage (with locked-in syndrome)

History
- Clarify if patient has had recent concussion with postconcussive symptoms.
- Recent alcohol or substance abuse
- H/o of diabetic hypoglycemia

Exam
- Neurologic exam

Testing
- Acute neuroimaging

Pitfalls
- Extremely uncommon syndrome, so rarely considered in the face of mild TBI.

Red Flags
- Individuals with any recent history or possible or probable TBI must be considered at high risk for second impact syndrome with new injury.
- Individuals who are slow to completely resolve after mild TBI must have a brain neuroimaging study (CT scan or MRI).

Treatment

Medical
- Acute Trauma Life Support

Exercises
- None

Modalities
- None

Surgical
- Emergent neurosurgical intervention

Consults
- None

Complications/side effects
- Death

Prognosis
- Poor

Helpful Hints
- Clinical deterioration (2–5 minutes) far more rapid than epidural hematoma (reaches fatal size in 30–60 min)

- An athlete with residual symptoms or neurologic signs from a brain injury *must not* participate in sports until all symptoms have resolved.

Suggested Reading
Cantu RC. Second-impact syndrome. *Clin Sports Med* 1998;17:37–44.

Concussion: Sports

Description
- Sports-related damage to the brain induced by the brain moving violently within the skull that results in transient, minor, mental status changes; mild TBI
- Simple concussions have symptoms that resolve in 7–10 days
- Complex concussions have symptoms that last > 10 days

Etiology
- Usually the result of rapid acceleration/deceleration of head with transient disruption of axonal activity
- Primarily reversible neurometabolic pathophysiology
- Usually not associated with macroscopic changes on CT scan; however, diffuse axonal injury (white matter tract hemorrhage) is the most common finding
- Magnetic resonance imaging (MRI) is the best modality to see acute abnormalities

Risk Factors
- Highest risk seen in football, hockey players and cheerleaders

Clinical Features
- While postconcussive symptoms are common after TBI, persistent symptoms and three or more symptoms are not.
- Research demonstrates that neurophysiologic abnormalities are worse in first 48 hours and rapidly return to normal baseline by 2 weeks postinjury.
- Symptoms are predominately physical in nature at onset of PCS but later progress to a more psychological presentation.
- Physical symptoms include headache, dizziness, fatigue, noise sensitivity, nausea, vomiting, light sensitivity, decreased sense of taste/smell, blurred vision, diplopia, tinnitus, and hearing loss and are typically present within the first 48 hours.
- Cognitive symptoms include memory deficits (especially short-term memory), difficulty concentrating, personality changes, and slowed information processing and are typically noticed within the first 2 weeks postinjury.
- Behavioral symptoms include irritability, poor judgment, restlessness, agitation, decreased libido, and impaired social interaction and may not be noticed for 4 weeks postinjury.
- Emotional symptoms include depression, anxiety, and lability.

Diagnosis

Differential diagnosis
- TBI severity is moderate or severe if initial Glasgow Coma Scale score is < 13, loss of consciousness is > 30 minutes or if any of the following seen on CT scan
  - Subdural hematoma
  - Epidural hematoma
  - Intracerebral hemorrhage
  - Subarachnoid hemorrhage
  - Cerebral contusions

History
- Identify specifics of injury and events/status surrounding time of injury
- If possible, verify injury specifics via emergency department and medical records, EMS run sheets, and witnesses.
- Prior concussion
- Preinjury drug or alcohol usage
- Use of helmet
- Identify sport-related prior injuries

Exam
- Mental status assessment
- Full neurologic exam
- Depression screen

Testing

- CT scanning is (by definition) normal, except in the case of "complicated mild TBI" where small amounts of subarachnoid hemorrhage may be seen.
- Neuropsychological assessment of general intellectual ability, perception, judgment, verbal, and constructive and executive functions
- Balance testing
- Advanced neuroimaging (MRI) if history, exam, initial testing, and symptoms are not congruous (see Assessment Scales: Concussion Grading)

Pitfalls

- Athletes may downplay injury specifics and symptoms to allow for early return to play

Red Flags

- Be aware of second impact syndrome; second concussion before symptoms of first have resolved.
- Be aware of cumulative effects of multiple concussions.

Treatment

Medical

- Acute management on the field consists of standard protocol.
  - ABCs—airway, breathing, circulation
  - Immobilization of the C-spine

Exercises

- Rapid return to play is encouraged, using Return to Play Guidelines

Modalities

- Cognitive assistive technology

Surgical

- N/A

Consults

- N/A

Complications/side effects

- Rare

Prognosis

- In all, 15% to 30% individuals will have persistent symptoms at 1 to 3 months, 3% at 1 year.
- Much higher return to work rates than moderate or severe brain injury

Helpful Hints

- Consideration for return to play should only be done if there are no residual neurological deficits, all postconcussive symptoms have resolved, and all testing that has been done (both imaging and neuropsychological testing) has returned to normal/baseline.
- Beware of second impact syndrome (see Concussion: Second Impact Syndrome, page 54)

Suggested Reading

Koh JO, Cassidy JD, Watkinson EJ. Incidence of concussion in contact sports: A systemic review of the evidence. *Brain Inj* 2003;17:901–917.

Powell JW, Barber-Foss KD. Traumatic brain injury in high school athletes. *JAMA* 1999;282:958–963.

Coordination Deficits

Description
- Coordination: the harmonious functioning of muscles or groups of muscles in the execution of movements
- Ataxia: jerky and inaccurate movement of either the trunk or extremities despite normal
- Strength and tone
- Dysmetria: the inability to accurately move an intended distance

Etiology
- Seen with all severities of TBI, worse with greater severity
- Most commonly seen with cerebellar involvement

Risk Factors
- Injuries that result in an impairment of special senses and somatosensory feedback to cerebellum

Clinical Features
- Difficulty in smoothly and precisely executing movements
- Increased time and effort required for functional tasks
- Increased likelihood of dropping/mishandling objects and falls
- May be associated with dysarthria
- Vermal (midline) cerebellar injury is more likely to result in truncal incoordination (ataxia), while para-vermal (lateral lobes) lesions are more likely to result in limb incoordination.

Diagnosis

Differential diagnosis
- Stroke/aneurysm/arteriovenous malformation
- Multiple sclerosis
- Brain tumor
- Myelopathy
- Peripheral neuropathy
- Acute intoxication
- Delirium tremens
- Intention tremor
- Hepatic encephalopathy
- Familial ataxia

History
- Identify prior tremor disorder
- Identify prior coordination deficits

Exam
- Perform complete cranial nerve, motor, sensory, tone, and deep tendon reflex examination
- Examine for dysdiadochokinesia (inability to perform rapid alternating movements)
- Examine for visual acuity and nystagmus
- Examine finger-to-nose and heel-to-shin testing
- Examine sitting and standing balance
- Evaluate gait

Testing
- Brain imaging to define etiology of brain injury
- Spine imaging if history consistent with spine trauma or motor/sensory examination localizes lower motor neuron–related weakness
- Electrophysiologic testing to clarify differential diagnosis (EEG for Todd paralysis, EMG for lower motor neuron disorder)

Pitfalls
- Increased tone or spasticity may limit ability to assess coordination.
- Weakened extremity may appear poorly coordinated despite intact cerebellum.

Red Flags
- Increasing incoordination

Treatment

Medical
- No proven medication effects

Exercises/rehabilitation
- Patterned movements to enhance coordination
- Speech services to enhance vocal clarity

- Weighted orthotics or utensils may improve coordination.
- Assistive devices are used to enhance stability.
- Constraint-induced movement therapy for upper extremity may be tried.
- Forced-use movement therapy, including body weight supported treadmill training for lower extremity
- Sensorimotor techniques to facilitate improved neurologic recovery and normal neurologic patterning, including those proposed by Bobath or Brunnstrom

Modalities
- None

Surgical
- No proven role for muscle transplantation

Consults
- Speech and language pathology for coordination deficits of speech or swallowing

Complications/side effects
- Falls

Prognosis
- Rate of recovery negatively correlated with initial incoordination

Helpful Hints
- Repetitive tasking appears to be the best proven intervention.

Suggested Reading
Neistadt ME. The effects of different treatment activities on functional fine motor coordination in adults with brain injury. *Am J Occup Ther* 1994;48(10):877–882.

Cranial Nerve Deficits—I (Anosmia)

Description
- Cranial nerve I (olfactory nerve) carries sensory information of smell.
- Olfactory nerve axons pass through the cribiform plate of the ethmoid bone and then synapse in the olfactory bulbs.
- The olfactory bulbs project to higher cortical areas of the brain that process the sense of smell: entorhinal cortex, hypothalamus, dorsal medical thalamic nucleus, and orbitofrontal cortex.
- Olfactory impairment seen in up to 33% of TBI cases.
- Anosmia: inability to smell
- Dysnosmia: impaired ability to smell
- Hyposmia: partial loss of ability to smell
- Parosmia: detecting smells in the absence of stimulus
- Cacosmia: awareness of a nonexistent noxious odor (as seen in preseizure aura)

Etiology
- Shearing of the olfactory nerve fibers as they cross the cribiform plate (via rotational forces or cribiform plate fractures)
- Compression of olfactory bulbs by secondary brain injury including edema, hemorrhage, contusion, abrasion
- Trauma to the orbital frontal or anterior temporal lobes
- May have delayed onset of symptoms due to scarring of tissues surrounding the cribiform plate

Risk Factors
- Orbitofrontal brain damage
- H/o cerebral spinal fluid rhinorrhea

Clinical Features
- Most commonly injured cranial nerve in mild TBI
- Higher incidence in moderate-severe head injuries
- Only 30% of patients are aware of their deficit.
- The more severe the injury, the more unlikely a patient will be aware of his deficit.
- Despite having partial anosmia, 70% can detect noxious stimuli like gasoline, paint thinner, smoke, motor oil, natural gas.

- Anosmia has been associated with problems in executive function and functional outcome.
  - Executive system impairments include inappropriate humor, inappropriate displays of sexuality, labile behaviors, desire for immediate gratification of needs, and disinhibition.
  - Anosmia leads to post-TBI employment problems as anosmics have higher rates of vocational disability even in the setting of normal intelligence and memory.

Diagnosis
Differential diagnosis
- Nasal edema due to trauma, upper respiratory tract infection, allergic sinusitis
- Chronic polyposis
- Seizures
- Olfactory hallucinations
- Injury to nasal cavity
- Anterior cranial fossa tumor
- Toxin exposure

History
- Difficulty detecting odors
- Food is tasteless.
- H/o cerebral spinal fluid rhinorrhea, frontal/occipital blows, frontal skull fractures

Exam
- Evaluate patency of nares
- University of Pennsylvania Smell Identification Test—40-item smell recognition test via scratch and sniff cards.

Imaging
- Olfactory encephalography
- Ethmoid CT to determine if fracture is present
- Perfusion SPECT imaging may demonstrate lesions involving frontal, temporal, and temporoparietal cortex (MRI may appear anatomically normal).
- Quantitative PET scan may demonstrate hypometabolism in the orbitofrontal cortex and/or medial temporal lobe.
- If parosmia is present, order EEG to assess for seizure activity.

Pitfalls

- Cognitive deficits may preclude definitive testing.
- Institutional bacterial colonization of the nares can alter smell.
- Weight loss poor nutrition due to the inability to enjoy food

Red Flags

- Olfactory auras may be associated with seizure activity.

Treatment

Medical

- No established effective treatment, initially observation

Rehabilitation

- Develop a routine with the patient that involves daily hygiene tasks, as patients may not be able to perceive body odor.
- Patient should be taught to date perishable items so that if an item's freshness is questionable, the date can be used to assess usability.
- Install smoke alarms on all floors of the house
- Teach patients to increase taste of food with spicing to encourage intake

Exercises

- None

Modalities

- None

Surgical

- Potential surgical exploration of cribriform plate fractures with scarring

Consults

- Otolaryngology

Complications/side effects

- Fractures to the cribriform plate, as well as surgical exploration of the region, are frequently associated with cerebrospinal fluid leakage from dural injury.

Prognosis

- Approximately one-third recover, one-third worsen, and one-third of patients have no change.
- Early recovery may be due to resolution of edema of smell pathways.

Helpful Hints

- In all, 40% of patients with history of CSF rhinorrhea experience anosmia.
- May see concomitant loss of appetite
- Patients may complain that food is tasteless
- Anosmia may serve as a unique marker for orbital frontal lobe executive functions.

Suggested Reading

Costanzo RM, Becker DFP. Sense of smell and taste disorders in head injury and neurosurgery patients. In: Meiselman HL, Rivlin RS, eds. *Clinical Management of Taste and Smell.* New York: Macmillan; 1986:565–578.

Section II: Conditions

Cranial Nerve Deficits—V, VII (Face)

Description
- Trigeminal nerve (cranial nerve V) supplies motor innervation to muscles of mastication and some smaller muscles of the face, general sensation anterior two-thirds of tongue, and facial sensation.
- Facial nerve (cranial nerve VII) supplies sensation to external ear and tympanic membrane, motor to muscles of facial expression, taste to anterior two-thirds of tongue, and visceral motor to lacrimal and salivary glands.

Etiology
- Trigeminal nerve injury may occur from orbit blowout fracture (especially V1 and V2 portions), superficial blow to face, transverse skull fractures, and cavernous sinus injury.
- Facial nerve injury may occur from temporal bone (most common) and petrous bone fractures, or an injury to the pons.
- The facial nerve is the second most commonly injured cranial nerve, after the olfactory nerve (CN I).
- A petrous bone fracture may result in a combined injury to cranial nerves VII and VIII. An injury at the level of the cranial nerve VII nucleus will likely also cause lateral rectus weakness (CN VI).

Risk Factors
- Transverse skull fractures (CN V)
- Cavernous sinus fractures (CN V)
- Temporal bone fractures (CN VII)
- Petrous bone fractures (CN VII)
- Pontine injury (CN VII)

Clinical Features
- Trigeminal nerve injury results in facial numbness, weakness of muscles of mastication, and you may see pain resulting from sensory neuropathy (trigeminal neuralgia).
- With trigeminal nerve injury, you will see sensory sparing of angle of jaw (supplied by upper cervical roots).

- Facial nerve injury results in ipsilateral weakness of the muscles of facial expression (eg, nasolabial fold, smile, forehead) and decreased sensation on the anterior two-thirds of the tongue.

Diagnosis

Differential diagnosis
- Upper motor neuron injury to nucleus of CN V or VII

History
- Preexisting deficits in CN V or VII

Exam
- For trigeminal nerve injury, assess for facial sensation (including corneal sensation) and test strength of muscles of mastication (although testing for masseter weakness may be difficult).
- For facial nerve injury, assess for inability to taste in anterior two-thirds of tongue, external ear sensation, dry eyes/dry mouth, forehead wrinkling (if present, but midfacial muscles weakened suggest UMN lesion, if absent a lower motor neuron injury), and presence of "crocodile tears" (while eating, tears develop instead of or with salivation, due to misguided nerve regeneration).
- Check extraocular movements to evaluate for CN VI dysfunction
- Balance and hearing tests to assess for injury to CN VIII

Testing
- Electromyography and nerve conduction studies of CN VII

Pitfalls
- Crocodile tears

Red Flags
- Worsening weakness of facial muscles acutely may suggest edema; cortisteroids and surgical consultation are indicated.

Treatment

Medical

- For trigeminal nerve injury, frequent eye irrigation to prevent corneal abrasion and anticonvulsants for trigeminal neuralgia.
- For facial nerve injury, topical lubricant to eyes of eyelid closure affected (in severe cases, operation to close lid may be indicated)
- For facial nerve, if delayed facial weakness, there may be facial nerve swelling. Start corticosteroids and consult otolaryngology for facial nerve decompression.

Exercises

- Focal strengthening exercises of select muscles

Modalities

- While poorly tolerated (due to pain), functional electrical stimulation to facial muscles may be used.

Surgical

- Surgical consult for possible CN XII to CN VII crossover

Consults

- Otolaryngology
- Ophthalmology

Complications/side effects

- Corneal irritation is a significant concern acutely after CN VII injury.

Prognosis

- Excellent for acute lower motor nerve injury at 3 months
- Worse prognosis for upper motor nerve injury (at nucleus level) compared to lower motor nerve injury

Helpful Hints

- The ability to wrinkle the forehead in the presence of midface muscle weakness indicated an upper motor neuron injury to the CN VII.
- Nontraumatic CN VII dysfunction is called Bell palsy.

Suggested Reading

Berol S. Cranial nerve dysfunction. *Phys Med Rehabil: State of the Art Rev* 1989;3(1):85–93.

Keane JR, Baloh RW. Post-traumatic cranial neuropathies. *Neurol Clin* 1992;10:849–867.

Cranial Nerve Deficits—X, XI, XII (Head and Neck)

Description

- Vagus nerve (cranial nerve X) provides motor innervation to the pharynx and soft palate, provides parasympathetic motor innervation to the trachea, bronchi, esophagus, and GI tract, slows heart rate, and provides sensory innervation to the pharynx, larynx, and thoraco-abdominal viscera.
- Spinal accessory nerve (cranial nerve XI) provides motor innervation to sternocleidomastoid and upper half of trapezius.
- Hypoglossal nerve (cranial nerve XII) provides motor innervation to intrinsic tongue muscles.

Etiology

- Vagus nerve injury results from blunt trauma from occipital condyle.
- Spinal accessory nerve injury results from blunt trauma to lateral neck.
- Hypoglossal nerve injury results from penetrating wounds to neck.

Risk Factors

- Trauma to the occipital condyle (CN X)
- Blunt trauma to lateral neck (CN XI)
- Penetrating wounds to the neck (CN XII)

Clinical Features

- Vagus nerve injury may result in dysphagia and aphonia.
- Spinal accessory nerve injury results in inability to turn head to opposite side and ipsilateral shoulder drooping.
- Hypoglossal nerve injury may result in dysarthria and/or dysphagia.

Diagnosis

Differential diagnosis

- Hemiparesis will result in shoulder weakness (CN XI)

History

- Preexisting difficulties with vision, hearing, or swallowing

Exam

- With vagus nerve injury, test gag reflex and palate elevation.
- With spinal accessory nerve injury, check head movements and the ability to raise shoulders.
- With hypoglossal nerve injury, check for tongue atrophy and/or fasciculations, and deviation of the tongue with protrusion.

Testing

- EMG testing for CN XI injury

Pitfalls

- Central injuries to the brainstem will have similar deficits as lower motor neuron injuries to CN X or XII.

Red Flags

- Worsening acute deficits from CN X, XI, or XII injuries may be evidence of ongoing hemorrhage from neck trauma.

Treatment

Medical

- None

Exercises

- For vagus nerve injuries, speech and language pathology for pharyngeal exercises
- For spinal accessory nerve injuries, strengthening to neck and shoulder muscles

Modalities

- For functional electrical stimulation to neck and shoulder muscles

Surgical

- Thyroplasty and arytenoids surgical adduction for high vagus nerve injuries
- Teflon, Gelfoam, or fat injection into vocal cord(s) for short-term approximation of vocal cords with vagus nerve injury
- With lower motor nerve hypoglossal nerve injury, surgical correction is recommended if poor recovery in 3 months.

Consults

- Otolaryngology
- Speech and language pathology

Complications/side effects

- Surgical procedures to vocal cords may result in acute edema with transient worsening.

Prognosis

- Recovery occurs in the first 3 to 6 months postinjury.
- Lower motor neuron injuries have a better prognosis for full recovery.

Helpful Hints

- With hypoglossal nerve injury, tongue deviation toward lesion indicates a peripheral (lower motor neuron) injury and tongue deviation away from lesion indicates a central (upper motor neuron) injury.

Suggested Reading

Berol S. Cranial nerve dysfunction. *Phys Med Rehabil: State of the Art Rev* 1989;3(1):85–93.
Keane JR, Baloh RW. Post-traumatic cranial neuropathies. *Neurol Clin* 1992;10:849–867.

Section II: Conditions

Cranial Nerve Deficits—III, IV, VI (Ocular Muscles)

Description
- Oculomotor nerve (CN III)
  - Nucleus arises paramedially in the midbrain.
  - Fibers penetrate dura at the cavernous sinus.
  - Passes through superior orbital fissure
  - Innervates medial rectus, superior rectus, inferior rectus, inferior oblique, and levator palpebrae muscle.
  - Parasympathetic fibers originating from the Edinger-Westphal nucleus course closely with the oculomotor nerve
- Trochlear nerve (CN IV)
  - Emerges from midbrain, enters cavernous sinus, and then innervates the contralateral superior oblique muscle (SOM)
  - SOM deviates the eye down and in.
  - Longest intracranial course of all the cranial nerves
  - Very slender connection to the brainstem
  - Damaged in up to 1.4% of TBIs
- Abducens nerve (CN VI)
  - Originates in pons, pierces dura lateral to sphenoid bone, enters cavernous sinus, passes through superior orbital fissure to innervate the lateral rectus muscle

Etiology
- Oculomotor nerve palsy
  - Injury can occur anywhere along its course; however, nerve is most commonly injured either where it penetrates the dura or by uncal herniation compression.
  - Correlated with subarachnoid hemorrhage and skull fractures
- Trochlear nerve palsy
  - Tends to occur after diffuse frontal or occipital impact causing sagittal forces to the brainstem
  - Cavernous sinus thrombosis
  - Unilateral lesions are usually caused by the nerve being compressed against the tentorium or damaged as it exits the brainstem.
- Abducens nerve palsy
  - Damage from trauma anywhere along its course
  - Hydrocephalus

Risk Factors
- Uncal herniation compression
- Diffuse frontal or occipital impact causing sagittal forces to the brainstem

Clinical Features
- Oculomotor nerve palsy
  - "Down and out" deviation of eye
  - Ptosis
  - Eye can only move laterally (lateral rectus intact)
  - Double vision
  - Absent accommodation
  - Pupillary dilation if complete lesion (parasympathetic fibers are damaged, leading to unopposed sympathetic stimulation)
- Trochlear nerve palsy
  - Vertical diplopia when looking downward (especially when walking down steps)
  - Improves with contralateral head tilt
  - Worsens with ipsilateral head tilt
  - Isolated lesions of the nucleus cause contralateral symptoms because the fibers decussate at the level of the brainstem.
  - Position of the eye may appear normal, as other unaffected ocular muscles compensate for the superior oblique dysfunction.
- Abducens nerve palsy
  - Eye deviated medially in complete lesion
  - Eye cannot be deviated laterally.
  - If damage is at the level of nucleus, will see evidence of facial nerve damage as these fibers loop around CN VI nucleus

Diagnosis

Differential diagnosis
- Cavernous sinus thrombosis
- Tumor
- Diabetic infarctions to the nerve
- Multiple sclerosis
- Meningitis

History
- Specific visual complaints

Exam

- Check extraocular movements
- Pupillary reaction
  - With an efferent injury to CN III, the affected pupil will not constrict with light shown into either eye. However, opposite pupil will constrict to light shone into affected eye.
- Eyelid elevation
- Check for accommodation
- Doll's-eyes maneuver if unconscious
- Bielschowsky head-tilt test for CN IV dysfunction: test is positive if there is further separation of images when head is tilted to the affected eye. Likewise, there is a reduction in diplopia when head is tilted toward unaffected eye.

Testing

- Imaging: CT or MRI
  - Precise localization of CN IV lesion is difficult, except in cases where there is obvious orbital or skull base trauma that likely affects the nerve in its peripheral course.
  - If midbrain contusion is suspected, MRI is the test of choice.

Pitfalls

- Cognitive deficits may preclude definitive testing.

Red Flags

- Fixed and dilated pupil due to oculomotor nerve compression may signify impending uncal herniation.

Treatment

Medical

- Neurolytic blockade to ipsilateral medial rectus in CN VI dysfunction

Exercises

- Eye muscle strengthening exercises have limited efficacy.

Modalities

- Patching to resolve diplopia
- Prism lenses to glasses to accommodate for muscle weakness

Surgical

- Strabismus surgery may be considered, but it is recommended to wait until maximal visual acuity is recovered.

Consults

- Ophthalmology
- Orthoptist

Complications/side effects

- Corrective surgery to rebalance eye musculature will initially result in difficulties in visual orientation and often diplopia that may take weeks to correct. In individuals with persistent cognitive deficits, these acute abnormalities may worsen the functional difficulties arising from these deficits.

Prognosis

- CN III: some improvement in function in 2 to 3 months, but often the recovery is incomplete.
- CN IV: Unpredictable recovery; 44% spontaneously recover.
- CN VI: Spontaneous resolution seen for 12% to 84% of cases. Prognosis better for unilateral cases.

Helpful Hints

- Oculomotor nerve palsy may be misdiagnosed in orbital blowout fractures. Check for infraorbital numbness, as this is not consistent with oculomotor nerve palsy.
- Dilation of both pupils indicates deep coma or death.

Suggested Reading

Keane JR, Baloh RW. Post-traumatic cranial neuropathies. *Neurol Clin* 1992;10:849–867.

Sabates NR, Gonce MA, Farris BK. Neuro-ophthalmological findings in closed head injury. *J Clin Neuro-ophthalmology* 1991;11:273–277.

Section II: Conditions

Cranial Nerve Deficits—II, VIII, IX (Special Senses)

Description
- Optic nerve (cranial nerve II) provides the sense of sight.
- Vestibulocochlear nerve (cranial nerve VIII) provides special sensory for hearing and equilibrium and balance
- Glossopharyngeal nerve (cranial nerve IX) provides sensation and taste to posterior one-third of tongue, soft palate and pharynx sensation, innervates chemoreceptors and baroreceptors from carotid body, provides motor innervation to stylopharyngeus and pharynx, and provides parasympathetic innervation to the parotid gland.

Etiology
- Optic nerve injury results from injury to globe or injury to the orbitofrontal lobe of the brain.
- Vestibulocochlear nerve results from temporal bone fracture.
- Vestibulocochlear nerve injury can occur with trauma to the jugular foramen.

Risk Factors
- The optic nerve is susceptible to primary (eg, globe injury) and secondary injury (eg, frontal lobe injury).
- Temporal bone fractures (CN VIII)
- Jugular foramen injury (CN VIII)

Clinical Features
- Optic nerve injury may result in complete monocular blindness (+ abnormal pupillary reflexes), partial monocular blindness or visual field deficits if injury at optic chiasm or more distal.
- Vestibulocochlear nerve injury may result in vertigo, tinnitus, and sensorineural hearing loss.
- Glossopharyngeal nerve injury may result in loss of taste over posterior tongue, decreased salivation, and mild dysphagia.

Diagnosis

Differential diagnosis
- Gray-matter injury along the visual pathways (temporal-parietal lobes) or visual cortex (occipital lobes) may resemble CN II injury.
- Damage to primary structures of eye (eg, cornea, lenses)
- Damage to the ear canal or tympanic membrane
- Central dysphagia

History
- Preexisting difficulties with vision, hearing, or swallowing

Exam
- With optic nerve injury, test papillary reaction to light, visual acuity, visual fields, and perform an ophthalmoscope exam to r/o retinal detachment.
- With vestibulocochlear nerve injury, look for mastoid ecchymosis acutely (Battle sign), otorrhea (hemorrhage from the ear), nystagmus elicited with extraocular movement, cold water calorics, or Dix-Hallpike maneuver, and a decline in hearing acuity as measured with Weber and Rinne Tests
- Otoscopic exam with CN VIII injury to evaluate tympanic membrane for tears or hemo-tympanium.
- With glossopharyngeal nerve injury, look for deviation of uvula to contralateral side, test for oropharyngeal sensation, and assess gag reflex.

Testing
- For CN VIII injury, look for nystagmus elicited with extraocular movement, cold water calorics, or Dix-Hallpike maneuver.
- For CN VIII injury, look for a decline in hearing acuity as measured with audiometry or with Weber/Rinne Tests.

Pitfalls
- It may be challenging to discern CN II injuries from gray-matter injury to the visual cortex in cognitively impaired individuals.

Red Flags
- Hemorrhage from ear (otorrhea) may signify temporal bone fracture.

Treatment

Medical
- With CN VIII injury, meclizine is discouraged due to sedation and possible deterrence of central adaptation.

■ If only CN IX involved, symptoms are usually limited and do not need treatment.

Exercises

■ Labyrinthine exercises to improve equilibrium with CN VIII injury

Modalities

■ Orthoptics, such as Fresnel lenses, are used for field deficits in CN II injury.
■ Hearing aids for deficits from CN VIII
■ For tinnitus from CN VIII injury, masking sound devices and biofeedback.

Surgical

■ If conductive hearing loss is present and does not spontaneously resolve, refer to otolaryngologist for possible surgery.

Consults

■ Otolaryngology
■ Neuro-ophthalmologist consultation

Complications/side effects

■ Orthoptic usage is often challenging for cognitively intact individuals and is especially difficult for individuals with persistent cognitive deficits.

Prognosis

■ CN II is direct extension of brain and will not regenerate.

Helpful Hints

■ Visual field deficits if optic nerve injury at optic chiasm or more distal
■ Transverse temporal bone fractures resulting in CN VIII injury will cause sensorineural hearing loss, and longitudinal temporal bone fractures usually cause mixed conductive / sensorineural hearing loss.

Suggested Reading

Sabates NR, Gonce MA, Farris BK. Neuro-ophthalmological findings in closed head injury. *J Clin Neuro-opthalmology* 1991;11:273–277.

Sismanus A. Post-concussive neuro-otological disorders. *Phys Med Rehabil: State of the Art Reviews* 1992;6(1):79–88.

Steinsapir KD. Traumatic optic neuropathy. *Curr Opin Ophthalmol* 1999;10(5):340–342.

Cranial/Skull Defects: Craniotomy/ Craniectomy/Cranioplasty

Description
- Craniotomy: any surgical opening of the skull
- Craniectomy: removal of portion of the skull
- Cranioplasty: surgery that corrects skull defects

Etiology
- Surgical procedure typically related to need to urgently relieve intracranial pressure from acute hydrocephalus

Risk Factors
- Acute, focal subdural, or interparenchymal hemorrhage

Clinical Features
- Craniotomy
  - Also known as a "burr hole"
  - An emergency craniotomy can be used to urgently diagnose and treat a rapidly expanding subdural hematoma.
  - Used for pressure monitors and drains. These sensors may also be used for oxygen monitoring and CSF analysis (lactate, neurotransmitters).
- Craniectomy
  - An emergency craniectomy can be used for rapidly expanding subdural hematomas that need to be evacuated.
  - Craniectomies (usually bifrontal) are occasionally done to control rising intracranial pressure despite absence of a mass lesion in patients who have failed medical therapy.
  - This procedure can result in delayed problems, with CSF dynamics that can lead to hydrocephalus; however, problems with cerebral hemodynamics tend to resolve after cranioplasty.
  - Patients may need external ventricular or subdural drains
- Cranioplasty
  - refers to repair of bony defects due to craniectomy or traumas.
  - May see improvement in neurological function after cranioplasty
  - May see improvement in symptoms including headaches, dizziness, irritability, and epilepsy
  - Goal of cranioplasty is cosmesis, protection of the brain, and restoration of intracranial pressure dynamics.
  - Can involve either bone grafts or synthetic plates (ie, titanium).
  - Replacement of bone removed at time of craniectomy is preferred. The bone can be frozen, freeze dried, or stored in subcutaneous pockets in the patient.
  - Autogenous bone reconstruction can be done but more difficult with very large bony defects.
  - Complications include subdural hematomas and infection.
  - Neurosurgeons frequently refer to cranial bone grafts as "bone flaps."
  - Prior to cranioplasty, skin expansion may be necessary via a subcutaneous inflatable tissue expander.

Red Flags
- Elevated risk for infection with surgical penetration of the dura
- Elevated risk for intraparenchymal hemorrhage with all intracranial procedures
- Elevated risk for seizure with surgical penetration of the dura

Treatment

Medical
- One week of anticonvulsant agent (phenytoin) recommended after any procedure that opens the dura

Exercises
- N/A

Modalities
- N/A

Surgical
- N/A

Consults
- N/A

Complications/side effects
- Localized edema is common after surgery and may result in transient worsening of clinical condition. Late bleeding is rare but is another cause of worsening.
- Subarachnoid scarring after surgery can also contribute to higher rates of hydrocephalus.

Prognosis
- Worse functional outcome in individuals who require intracranial procedures

Helpful Hints
- Some clinicians feel that functional improvements arise after cranioplasty, although no research to support.
- Minimum of 6 weeks postcraniectomy before cranioplasty should be performed

Suggested Reading

Rish BL, Dillon JD, Meirowksy AM. Cranioplasty: A review of 1030 cases of penetrating injury. *Neurosurgery* 1979;4:381–385.

Section II: Conditions

Deep Venous Thrombosis

Description
- Thrombi in deep veins of pelvis, upper or lower extremities
- 10%–20% incidence upon admission to inpatient rehabilitation

Etiology
- Endothelial injury in setting of hypercoagulability initiates a coagulation mechanism.

Risk Factors
- Paralysis
- Immobility (especially protracted coma)
- Orthopedic surgery for concomitant body trauma
- Sepsis
- Prior history of deep venous thrombosis (DVT)
- Advanced age
- Congestive heart failure
- Obesity
- Myocardial infarction
- Malignancy
- Pregnancy
- Oral contraceptive use
- Smoking

Clinical Features
- Pain, edema, erythema are most common symptoms; however, these classic symptoms are present in only one-third of cases.
- Leg circumference discrepancy
- Prominent superficial veins

Diagnosis

Differential diagnosis
- Dependent edema
- Heterotopic ossification
- Occult fracture
- Varicose veins
- Superficial thrombophlebitis
- Achilles tendonitis
- Ruptured Baker cyst
- Cellulitis
- Lymphedema
- Arterial insufficiency
- Hematoma

History
- Family history of hypercoagulable state
- History of spontaneous abortion (related to antiphospholipid antibody syndrome)

Exam
- Physical exam techniques are of limited diagnostic value in detection of DVT.
- May see pain with dorsiflexion of ipsilateral foot in calf DVT—Homan sign

Testing
- Venous duplex ultrasonography
  - Consider using as screening tool
- Sensitive for proximal DVT but not distal DVT
- Interpretation dependent on skill and experience
- Gold standard—contrast venography
- Contraindicated in contrast allergy
- D-dimer–sensitive but not specific
- May be useful screening tool to exclude the likelihood of DVT
- False positives seen in trauma (first 6 weeks), fracture, surgery, sepsis, disseminated intravascular claudication

Pitfalls
- Less than one-third of DVT will present with typical symptoms.
- Risk of upper extremity DVT is often overlooked but seems to be as high as lower extremity.

Red Flags
- Acute shortness of breath, hemoptysis, tachycardia, and/or unexplained anxiety are common symptoms of PE.

Treatment

Medical
- Preventative therapy
  - Compressions devices
  - Graduated compression stocking (GCS) decrease incidence of DVT
  - Can be used concomitantly with other preventative treatments
  - Intermittent pneumatic compression—increases venous blood flow and systemic fibrinolytic activity

- Sequential compression devices are more effective than devices that compress leg uniformly.
- If initiated > 12 hours after trauma, screening studies should be considered to avoid compression of a newly formed DVT.
- May have increased efficacy when used in combination with graduated compression stockings
- May exacerbate agitation
- Usually cannot be used in lower extremity trauma
- Complications include chronic edema, propagation of clot above filter, filter fracture, filter migration, and venous wall perforation.
- Medications
- Low-molecular-weight heparin (LMWH) for moderate to severe risk of DVT; recommended prophylaxis for the acute period of care after TBI (2–6 weeks). May be started at 72 hours postintracranial bleeding.
- Warfarin is effective prophylactic agent if INR maintained between 2 and 3, but maintaining therapeutic level is extremely difficult.
- Unfractionated heparin (UFH)—effective for mild to moderate risk of thromboembolism but less effective for severe risk. Not first-line recommendation.
- Aspirin has little prophylactic benefit.
- Inferior Vena Cava (IVC), Greenfield, or Bird's Nest Filter
- Inappropriate for prophylaxis, but may be used in patients unable to be initially anticoagulated to reduce the risk for pulmonary embolus.
■ Treatment
- If no contraindication to anticoagulation, proximal DVTs are treated with UFH or therapeutic dosing of LMWH (Enoxaparin 1 mg/kg subcutaneous twice daily). May be started at 72 hours postintracranial bleeding.
- With use of UFH, goal PTT in first 24 hours is 1.5× normal.
- UFH can be administered intravenously or subcutaneously.
- Initial SQ dose is 30,000 twice daily and adjusted to therapeutic international normalized ration.
- Fondaparinux is a useful alternative in patients who cannot tolerate heparin.
- Warfarin usage follows initial heparin therapy, which should continue for 5 days initially.

- Continue for 3 months in DVT and 6 months for PE.
- IVC filter may be indicated in patients at high risk for DVT and in whom anticoagulation is contraindicated, or to help prevent PE; however, IVCs do not decrease incidence of DVT.

Exercises
■ When to resume exercise therapy after the diagnosis of DVT has not been definitively established; however, a return to full activity 24–48 hours after full anticoagulation has been advocated.

Modalities
■ None

Surgical
■ Interventional radiology or vascular surgery for IVC filter in individuals with DVT who have contraindications for full anticoagulation

Consults
■ Hematology if coagulopathy suspected

Complications/side effects
■ Watch for heparin-induced thrombocytopenia; monitor platelet counts 3 days after initiating treatment.

Prognosis
■ May lead to postphlebitic syndrome, recurrent DVT, and pulmonary embolism (PE), with an increased incidence in undertreated or untreated DVT
■ Postphlebitic syndrome marked by swelling, pain, induration, and venous claudication that can lead to disability

Helpful Hints
■ No set guidelines for timing of initiation of UFH or LMWH in patients with intracranial hemorrhage
■ Treatment of calf and upper extremity DVTs is controversial.
■ Pulmonary embolism has a 30% mortality, if left untreated.

Suggeste d Reading
Cifu DX, Kaelin DL, Wall BE. Deep venous thrombosis: Incidence on admission to a brain injury rehabilitation program. *Arch Phys Med Rehabil* 1996;77:1182–1185.

Section II: Conditions

Dementia and Traumatic Brain Injury

Description

- Dementia after TBI will present the same as in other causes, with chronic deterioration of mental function that includes memory, personality, behavior, attention, language, and abstract thought.
- The age at onset and/or rapidity of symptoms may be accelerated with concomitant TBI, a past h/o TBI with and without a genetic predisposition, or a history of multiple TBIs.

Etiology

- The specific relationship between dementia and TBI is not well elucidated.
- The rapid deterioration of dementia symptoms seen with an acute TBI is related to the limited neurologic reserve from underlying dementia.
- A 10× higher risk in the development of Alzheimer dementia is seen in individuals with a history of TBI and the APOE-epsilon 4 allele.
- Multiple TBIs (including mild) may predispose an individual to early onset dementia; however, the pathophysiology and relative risk are not well known.

Risk Factors

- Apolipoprotein E4 biomarker has been associated with a higher incidence of developing Alzheimer dementia after TBI.
- Possibly carriers of the APOE-epsilon 4 allele, which retards neural repair after trauma
- Multiple brain injuries (of any severity) may predispose to or result in dementia.

Clinical Features

- Memory deficits
- Deficiency in abstract thinking
- Deficits in calculation
- Loss of good judgment
- Personality changes
- Hallucinations
- Delusions

Diagnosis

Differential diagnosis

- Normal pressure hydrocephalus
- Depression
- Vascular dementia
- Hypothyroidism
- Neurosyphilis
- Substance-induced cognitive impairment
- Frontotemporal dementia
- Delirium
- Prion disease

History

- Initial insidious memory loss
- Slowly progressive behavioral changes
- May see language dysfunction
- Problems with activities of daily living
- Full social history, including alcohol intake
- Family history of dementia

Exam

- Cognitive assessment
- Gait assessment to assess for parkinsonism, vascular dementia, normal pressure hydrocephalus
- Full neurologic exam

Testing

- Laboratory evaluation of complete blood count, Vitamin B12 levels, thyroid stimulating hormone, rapid plasma reagent (RPR), liver function tests
- HIV testing for patients at risk
- Neuropsychological testing
- CT scan or MRI
- EEG if dementia presents with myoclonus—evaluate for prion disease

Pitfalls

- Dementia will manifest with progressive decline in deficits, while TBI has static deficits.

Red Flags

- Worsening memory deficits, especially long-term memory, may be indicative of dementing process.

Treatment

Medical

- Identify and treat modifiable or reversible causes of cognitive dysfunction.
- Treat depression if present.
- Acetylcholinesterase inhibitors for mild to moderate dementia
  - Rivastigmine tablets or transdermal patch
  - Donezepil
- N-methyl-D-aspartate antagonists for moderate to severe dementia
  - Memantadine

Exercises

- Regular aerobic exercise important in optimizing vascular health of brain.

Modalities

- Cognitive assistive technology

Surgical

- None

Consults

- Neuropsychology, to help differentiate dementia from pseudodementia

Complications/side effects

- None

Prognosis

- Progressive condition
- Medications do not slow course of disease.
- Most common cause of death is pneumonia.

Helpful Hints

- There is usually a discrepancy between a history obtained from the patient and the family, due to lack of insight on the part of the patient.

Suggested Reading

Jellinger KA. Head injury and dementia. *Curr Opinion Neurol* 2004;17:719–723.

Section II: Conditions

Depression

Description
- Altered psychomotor activity, classically defined as the presence of five of nine vegetative signs

Etiology
- Complex neurochemical alterations affecting the brain
- May also be due to abnormalities of the hypothalamic-pituitary axis
- Associated with metabolic abnormalities in the ventro- and dorsolateral prefrontal cortex and the anterior cingulate gyrus

Risk Factors
- High perceived stress
- Previous history of depression
- Family history of depression

Clinical Features
- Affects approximately 25%–60% of patients with TBI
- Vegetative signs include
  - Depressed mood
  - Difficulty with concentration
  - Insomnia
  - Hypersomnia
  - Difficulty with short-term memory
  - Loss of interest in once pleasurable activities
  - Psychomotor agitation, sometimes psychomotor retardation
  - Suicidal ideation
  - Loss of appetite
  - Delusions/hallucinations

Diagnosis

Differential diagnosis
- Normal bereavement
- Endocrine disorder: hypothyroidism, hypoadrenalism, hyperadrenalism
- Severe anemia
- Dysthymia: minor depression that is prolonged
- Cyclothymia: minor depression that cycles with hypomania
- Bipolar disorder: attacks of major depression and mania

History
- Assess sleep hygiene.
- Assess family history.
- Assess for hallucinations/delusions.
- Assess suicidal ideation.
- Assess use of alcohol/drugs.
- Assess for symptoms/signs of mania.
- For diagnosis patient needs to have five of the following for at least 2 weeks with noted disturbance in function: depressed mood, loss of pleasure and interest in activities, significant weight loss, insomnia or hypersomnia, agitation or retardation, fatigue or loss of energy, feelings of worthlessness or guilt, loss of concentration, recurrent thoughts of death or suicide.

Exam
- Full neurologic exam
- Cognitive assessment
- Behavioral assessment
- Depression scale

Testing
- Endocrine evaluation includes TSH, fasting AM cortisol, and sex hormone levels.

Pitfalls
- Depressive symptoms may overlap with those of post-concussive syndrome.

Red Flags
- Suicidal ideation

Treatment

Medical
- Review side effect profile before choosing medication.

- Psychotherapy
- Cognitive behavioral therapy
- Phototherapy

Surgical
- None

Consults
- Psychiatry, if resistant to treatment or suicidal

Complications/side effects
- Antidepressant medication often reduce appetite, so close monitoring of oral intake is warranted for the first 2–4 weeks after beginning or increasing medication dosing.

Prognosis
- Typically resolves in 6–12 months, but recurrence is likely without treatment

Helpful Hints
- Pseudodementia cerebri is the term for depression in the older adult that manifests as dementia.
- Presence or development of manic episodes during depression treatment, including delusions of grandeur or flight of ideas, may indicate bipolar disease.

Suggested Reading
Jorge RE, Robinson RG, Moser D, Tateno A, Crespo-Facorro B, Arndt S. Major depression following traumatic brain injury. *Arch Gen Psychiatr* 2004;61:42–50.

Section II: Conditions

Disinhibition

Description
- Disinhibition is a reduced capacity to edit or manage immediate impulsive response.
- Disinhibition is a common symptom following a physical injury to the brain, particularly to the frontal lobe. It may also be as a result of delirium, mania, alcohol, or drugs.

Etiology
- Frontal lobe injury, including frontotemporal and orbitotemporal regions

Risk Factors
- Injury to the frontal lobe
- Preinjury behavioral control issues
- Alcohol or illicit drug use

Clinical Features
- Disinhibition affects motor, instinctual, emotional, cognitive, and perceptual aspects with signs and symptoms similar to the diagnostic criteria for mania.
- Hypersexuality, hyperphagia, and aggressive outbursts are indicative of disinhibited instinctual drives.
- Typically improves with improving cognitive awareness

Diagnosis

Differential diagnosis
- Acute intoxication
- Delirium
- Mania
- Temporal lobe epilepsy

History
- H/o behavioral dyscontrol (eg, mania)
- H/o alcohol or illicit drug use

Exam
- Standard general physical examination
- Standard TBI examination

Testing
- Neuropsychological testing

Pitfalls
- Patients may commit inappropriate behaviors (eg, illegal activity) or alienate family and treatment staff, which makes future care difficult.

Red Flags
- Marked swings in behavior may suggest alternative etiology (eg, intoxication, epilepsy).

Treatment

Medical
- Antiepileptic agents (eg, valproic acid, carbamazepine) are good first-line agents.
- Selective serotonin reuptake inhibitors appear to have some efficacy.
- Lithium is effective, but potential risks limit usage.

Exercises/rehabilitation
- Behavioral management and modification are used in all settings.

Modalities
- N/A

Surgical
- N/A

Consults
- Psychiatry

Complications/side effects
- Patients with disinhibition are at high risk for unsafe behavior (eg, driving, substance use, police).

Prognosis

- Disinhibition is a common finding early after moderate and severe TBI, but typically improves in the initial 3–6 months. While far less common after mild TBI, it also typically improves by 3–6 months postinjury.
- Unlikely to improve spontaneously if persists past 6 months; however, medication and behavioral strategies are often successful.

Helpful Hints

- Patients with persistent disinhibition after TBI are likely to have significant difficulty with successfully reintegrating into their social and vocational situations.

Suggested Reading

Kim E. Agitation, aggression, and disinhibition syndromes after traumatic brain injury. *Neurorehabil* 2002;17(4):297–310.

Dizziness

Description
- Dizziness may include lightheadedness, presyncope, being unsteady, loss of balance, or vertigo.
- Balance is the maintenance of bodily equilibrium or stability.
- Vertigo is the illusion of movement.
- Presyncope is most often described as feeling lightheaded or faint. Presyncope does not result from primary central nervous system pathology.

Etiology
- Peripheral causes
- Benign paroxysmal positional vertigo (BPPV): displacement of crystal structures in semicircular canals
- Labyrinthine concussion
- CN VIII palsies: temporal bone fractures that damage inner ear or CN VIII
- Perilymphatic fistula—middle and inner ear boundary damaged
- Central causes
  - Trauma to brain stem
  - Trauma to the cerebellum
  - Posttraumatic migraines

Risk Factors
- Temporal bone fractures

Clinical Features
- BPPV
  - Vertigo and imbalance provoked by movement of the head
- Labyrinthine concussion
  - Hearing loss and vertigo
  - Sudden onset after head trauma
  - No fracture of temporal bone
- Perilympathic fistula
  - Sudden sensorineural hearing loss, vertigo, tinnitus

Diagnosis

Differential diagnosis
- Autonomic neuropathy
- Meniere's disease
- Labyrinthitis
- Cardiovascular etiologies, including vertebrobasiliar insufficiency
- Parkinson disease

History
- Premorbid history of dizziness
- Neurologic history

Exam
- Full neurologic exam
- Dix-Hallpike maneuver

Testing
- Audiometric testing
- Electronystamography
- Rotary chair
- Postural control assessment (computerized posturography)

Pitfalls
- Testing maneuvers, such as the Hallpike-Dix, often result in acute worsening of symptoms.

Red Flags
- Associated symptoms of confusion and/or incontinence, suggestive of hydrocephalus

Treatment

Medical
- The following are commonly used; however, they are not typically recommended (especially in the acute phase) due to negative cognitive effects and a delay in the natural recovery of the brain.
- Antihistamines
  - Meclizine
  - Promethazine

- Anticholinergics
  - Scopolamine
- Benzodiazepines
  - Diazepam
  - Lorazepam

Exercises

- BPPV
  - Canalith repositioning maneuvers
  - Liberatory technique (repeated and rapid movements of the head/body to recreate the dizziness) is used by physical therapists and otolaryngologists to extinguish symptoms.
- Gait instability
  - Exercises to enhance vestibular adaptation
  - Exercises to foster alternative mechanisms of gaze stability
- Postural instability
  - Exercises that involve varied sensory conditions including somatosensory changes, visual changes, and vestibular changes

Modalities

- None

Surgical

- Repair of perilymphatic fistula if present
- Temporal bone fracture repair

Consults

- Otolaryngology
- Neurosurgery

Complications/side effects

- Patients are often reluctant to undergo all aspects of treatment, especially that involving symptom recreation.

Prognosis

- Resolution of symptoms in >95% of patients in the first month postinjury.
- Improvements are most likely in first 6 months after injury.

Helpful Hints

- Comprehensive vestibular retraining programs address the multiple aspects of subacute and chronic dizziness that may be needed to optimize recovery.

Suggested Reading

Shepard NT, Clendaniel RA, Ruckenstein M. Balance and dizziness. In: Zasler ND, Katz DI, Zafonte RD, eds. *Brain Injury Medicine*. New York: Demos; 2007:491–510.

Section II: Conditions

Dysarthria

Description

- A motor speech disorder where the muscles of the mouth, face, and respiratory system may become weak, move slowly or spastically, or not move at all, resulting in speech that is characteristically slurred, slow, and difficult to produce (difficult to understand).
- The person with dysarthria may also have problems controlling the pitch, loudness, rhythm, and voice qualities of speech.

Etiology

- Injury to the brainstem

Risk Factors

- Severe TBI

Clinical Features

- "Slurred" speech
- Speaking softly or barely able to whisper
- Slow rate of speech
- Rapid rate of speech with a "mumbling" quality
- Limited tongue, lip, and jaw movement
- Abnormal intonation (rhythm) when speaking
- Changes in vocal quality ("nasal" speech or sounding "stuffy")
- Hoarseness
- Breathiness
- Drooling or poor control of saliva
- Chewing and swallowing difficulty

Diagnosis

Differential diagnosis

- Degenerative diseases such as Parkinson, Huntington, and Lou Gehrig disease/amyotrophic lateral sclerosis, multiple sclerosis, and cerebral palsy
- Excessive use of alcohol or drugs
- Long-term use or some medications
- Stuttering

History

- H/o substance abuse
- H/o neuroleptic medication use
- H/o schizophrenia
- H/o of Parkinson, Huntington, and Lou Gehrig disease/ALS, multiple sclerosis, and cerebral palsy
- H/o stuttering

Exam

- Standard general physical examination
- Standard TBI examination

Testing

- Modified barium swallow
- Flexible endoscopic evaluation of swallowing

Pitfalls

- Patients may reduce verbal output when dysarthria limits their understandability, thereby delaying recovery.

Red Flags

- Dysarthria, particularly when associated with a "wet" vocal quality, may be associated with dysphagia.

Treatment

Medical

- None

Exercises/rehabilitation

- Vocalization exercises
- Forced-use programs may play a role in early recovery.

Modalities

- Augmentative communication devices may be beneficial with severe dysarthria, although caution must be taken to encourage vocalization also.

Surgical

- None

Consults

- Speech language pathology
- Otolaryngology

Complications/side effects

- Association between dysphagia and dysarthria will increase risk for oral motor dysfunction, with resultant pocketing of food, drooling, and aspiration pneumonia.

Prognosis

- Improved outcome with unilateral dysarthrias related to motor weakness compared to spastic or cerebellar dysarthrias
- Typical recovery in the initial 3–6 months postinjury.

Helpful Hints

- Occasionally, regional dialects and vocal patterns may be interpreted as dysarthria.

Suggested Reading

Sarno M, Levin HS. Speech and language disorders after closed head injury. In: Darby JK, ed. *Speech Evaluation in Neurology: Adult Disorders*. New York: Grune and Stratton; 1985:323–339.

Dysphagia

Description
- Dysphagia is defined as difficulty swallowing and may include difficulties due to congenital abnormalities, structural abnormalities, or neuromuscular control of swallow.
- Neurogenic dysphagia may result from abnormalities in any of the three stages of swallowing: oral phase, pharyngeal phase, or esophageal phase.

Etiology
- Neurogenic dysphagia may be due to a cerebral or brainstem lesion.
- Brainstem lesions may directly affect the cranial nerves involved in swallowing (CN IX and X).
- Behavioral and cognitive deficits may also affect the swallowing process.

Risk Factors
- Initial intubation for TBI
- Traumatic/urgent intubation
- Tracheostomy
- Oropharyngeal spasticity or myoclonus

Clinical Features
- Coughing
- Choking
- Pain with swallowing
- "Wet" vocal quality
- Pocketing of food (especially, with unawareness)
- Weight loss
- Aspiration pneumonitis/pneumonia

Diagnosis

Differential diagnosis
- Preexisting or posttraumatic structural abnormalities of esophagus and trachea
- Psychogenic dysphagia (phagophobia)
- Painful swallowing (odynophagia)
- Globus pharyngis ("lump in one's throat")

History
- History of swallowing dysfunction
- History of weight loss

Exam
- Palpate hyoid bone, thyroid cartilage, and cricoid cartilage for any abnormalities
- Inspect oral cavity for secretions
- Cranial nerve testing
- Gag reflex
- Phonation

Testing
- Bedside swallowing evaluations are often used but have not been demonstrated to be reliable.
- Modified barium swallow testing (videofluorography) is the gold standard test.
- Fiberoptic endoscopic evaluation of swallowing (FEES) is a real-time observation of swallowing. Limited viewing of actual swallow limits utility.
- Delayed or absent swallowing reflex, aspiration, and oral phase dysfunction are the most common abnormalities found on videofluoroscopy

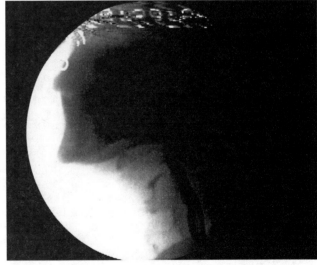

Lateral radiographic view of the oral cavity and pharynx at mid swallow in a patient post brain injury. The airway should be completely closed at this time but there is penetration and aspiration present. (With permission from Zasler ND, Katz DI, Zafonte RD. *Brain Injury Medicine: Principles and Practice.* New York: Demos; 2007.)

Pitfalls

- Radiation exposure with videofluorography
- FEES has two main limitations: (a) cannot visualize oral and esophageal swallowing phases and (b) does not evaluate the initial elevation of the larynx or contraction of the pharynx during the pharyngeal phase.
- Silent aspiration occurs in > 10% of dysphagia.

Red Flags

- Recurrent aspiration pneumonia (or fever of unknown origin) is a common indicator of dysphagia.

Treatment

Medical

- None

Exercises/rehabilitation

- Oral sensory training: cold and sour stimuli may improve timing of pharyngeal swallow.
- Electrical stimulation of anterior cervical strap muscles
- Suck-swallow exercises may improve bolus propulsion
- Laryngeal exercises include sustaining the sound "ee" and by swallowing with effort.
- Shaker exercise: while supine, isotonic-isometric neck flexion exercises are performed to strengthen the anterior suprahyoid muscles, which may facilitate upper esophageal sphincter opening during swallowing.
- Chopped or pureed solid foods that allow better bolus control during oral phase
- Thickened liquids for better control in the oral cavity and pharynx
- Chin tuck
- If unilateral pharyngeal weakness, turn head to weak side to force bolus over to the strong side.
- Neck extension to assist oral clearance when tongue movement is ineffective.
- Supraglottic swallow: patient holds breath prior to swallow to close off vocal cords.
- Effortful swallow: patient is instructed to swallow hard, which increases tongue movement and propels bolus during pharyngeal phase.
- Mendelsohn maneuver: patient is instructed to prolong contraction of suprahyoid muscles to help pharyngeal clearance.

Modalities

- Functional electrical stimulation (VitalStim) may be used to enhance neuromuscular control of swallow.

Prosthetics/orthotics

- Palatal augmentation prosthesis
- Palatal lift prosthesis can elevate the soft palate, which improves bolus propulsion.
- One-way speaking valves in patient with tracheostomies allow for cough and subsequent clearing of airway when aspiration occurs.

Surgical

- When dysphagia is severe and chronic, a permanent tracheostomy with laryngectomy may be necessary to completely separate the airway from the food passageway.
- Pharyngeal bypass with gastrostomy

Consults

- Speech language pathology

Complications/side effects

- Aspiration pneumonitis/pneumonia
- Gastrostomy tubes do not fully prevent aspiration.

Prognosis

- 75%–94% of individuals with TBI can eventually feed orally.

Helpful Hints

- Gag reflex does not predict against aspiration.
- "Wet vocal quality" is the most common physical finding.
- One-third of healthy adults have unilateral or bilateral absence of the gag reflex.
- Monitor for dehydration while a patient is on thickened liquids, especially when also taking diuretics.

Suggested Reading

Cherney LR, Halper AS. Swallowing problems in adults with traumatic brain injury. *Semin Neurol* 1996;16(4):349–353.

Emotional Lability

Description
- Type of agitated behavior, also known as affective lability, pathologic emotionalism, pseudobulbar affect, or emotional incontinence
- Pathologic display of emotion that is incongruous with an individual's actual mood
- Occurs in about 5% of patients

Etiology
- Unclear

Risk Factors
- Widespread cerebral pathology that is bilateral and involves the corticobulbar tracts

Clinical Features
- Increased readiness to laugh or cry
- Excessive laughing or crying that is often without associated feelings of happiness or sadness
- No voluntary control over extent or duration of episodes
- Recovery can be as rapid as onset.
- Crying is more commonly seen than laughter.
- Symptoms often occur in response to mild triggers.
- Symptoms can vary from mild to severe to socially disabling.
- Patients have insight into their illness and find their emotional lability distressing.
- Associated with intellectual impairment

Diagnosis

Differential diagnosis
- Emotional lability is also seen in
  - Cerebrovascular accident
  - Multiple sclerosis
  - Amyotrophic lateral sclerosis
  - Epilepsy
  - Dementia
- Depression

History
- History of prior neurologic illness
- History of depression

Exam
- Standard general physical examination
- Standard TBI examination

Pitfalls
- Depression may manifest with emotional lability.

Red Flags
- Worsening symptoms may be a sign of concomitant diagnosis (eg, depression).

Treatment

Medical
- SSRIs are typically first-line (fluoxetine is most studied).
- Avanir (first-in-class dual action glutamate inhibitor) has also been advocated.
- Levodopa
- Tricyclic antidepressants

Exercises
- Cognitive behavioral therapy

Surgical
- None

Consults
- Psychiatry

Complications/side effects

- Antidepressant medication often reduce appetite, so close monitoring of oral intake is warranted for the first 2–4 weeks after beginning or increasing medication dosing.

Prognosis

- Unknown

Helpful Hints

- Elements of emotional lability may be measured with the Agitated Behavior Scale.

Suggested Reading

Rao V, Lyketsos C. Neuropsychiatric sequelae of traumatic brain injury. *Psychosomat* 2000;41:95–103.

Executive Function Impairment

Description
- Cognitive process that is responsible for planning, abstract thinking, decision making, judgment, and regulation of attention
- Requires coordination of multiple cognitive processes to organize information
- Includes social cognition and motivational processes

Etiology
- Injury to the prefrontal cortex
- Dorsolateral prefrontal cortex mediates abstract thinking, planning, and working memory
- Medial prefrontal cortex mediates motivational and attention processes.
- Orbitofrontal lesions result in disinhibition, emotional lability, and insensitivity to the needs of others.

Risk Factors
- TBI associated with acceleration/deceleration forces leading to shearing and impact against the irregular skull base.

Clinical Features
- Disturbances of executive functioning usually become evident when an individual is required to deal with novel situations.
- Difficulty with tasks that require divided or alternating attention
- Inability to recognize other people's reactions to behavior
- May appear to be "high functioning" but have persistent social and vocational disabilities (eg, job loss, marital discord)
- Apathy (abulia)
- Disinhibition
- Emotional lability
- Lack of motivation
- Diminished social involvement

Diagnosis

Differential diagnosis
- Chronic alcohol use
- Depression
- Centrally acting medications
- Parkinson disease
- Premorbid executive functioning dysfunction (obsessive compulsive disorder, schizophrenia)

History
- Premorbid mental illness

Exam
- Mental status examination focused on abstract thinking, decision making, judgment, and attention
- Testing for frontal release signs

Testing
- Paced Auditory Serial Addition Test (working memory)
- Trail Making (divided attention and sequencing) Test
- Wisconsin Card Sorting Test
- Category Test (abstract thinking)

Pitfalls
- Behavioral dysfunction (stress disorder, anxiety, depression) or pain will impact executive functioning.

Red Flags
- Worsening of executive functioning after TBI may be a sign of acute process (edema, seizures) or a nonbrain injury cause (behavioral, medication, pain, secondary gain).

Treatment

Medical
- Limited efficacy with medications; however, dopaminergic drugs and amantadine may be considered

Exercises
- Goal management training
- Emotional self-regulation strategies

Modalities
- None

Surgical
- None

Consults
- Neuropsychology

Complications/side effects
- None

Prognosis
- Commonly seen after TBI with good resolution in most, related to severity
- Poor prognosis if little or slow recovery by 6 months

Helpful Hints
- An assessment of executive functioning during stressful settings (eg, at work) may be necessary to identify difficulties in highly functioning patients.

Suggested Reading

Eslinger PJ. Conceptualizing, describing, and measuring components of executive function. In: Lyon GR, Krasnegor NA, eds. *Attention, Memory, and Executive Function.* Baltimore, MD: Paul H. Brookes; 1996:367–396.

Levine B, Robertson IH, Clare L, Carter G. Rehabilitation of executive function: An experimental-clinical validation of goal management training. *J Int Neuropsychol Soc* 2000;6(3):299–312.

Gait (Ambulation) Dysfunction

Description
- Gait is a complex functional task that may be affected by abnormalities of any of its components, including strength, sensation, proprioception, balance, and special senses.
- Etiology
- Ambulation is affected by disorders of balance, coordination, strength, cognition, sensation, and vision.
- Non-TBI–related issues can include musculoskeletal injury, arthritides, weakness, pain, and environmental issues.

Risk Factors
- Disorders of ambulation are highly correlated with injury severity, initial gait impairment, and increased age.

Clinical Features
- Gait disorders include hemiplegic (foot drop with steppage gait), spastic (ankle plantar flexion with knee genu recurvatum, hip hiking with circumduction), ataxic (wide-based), and parkinsonian (shuffling, festinating with limited arm swing, en bloc turns).
- Falls, with and without injury, may be the end product of gait abnormalities.

Diagnosis

Differential diagnosis
- Lower extremity arthritis
- Parkinson disease
- Normal pressure hydrocephalus (NPH)
- Benign paroxysmal positional vertigo
- Inner ear (labyrinthine) concussion with otolith dislodgement
- Labyrinthitis
- Vertebrobasiliar artery insufficiency
- Orthostatic hypotension
- Peripheral neuropathy
- Posterior column (spinal cord) damage

- Central acting medications
- Alcohol intoxication/Korsakoff syndrome

History
- Prior gait or lower extremity abnormalities
- Other Parkinson disease symptoms (motor freezing, shuffling gait, tremor, mask facies)
- Other NPH symptoms (worsening cognition and/or incontinence)

Exam
- Perform complete cerebellar, basal ganglia, cranial nerve, motor, sensory, tone, and deep tendon reflex examination
- Examine sitting and standing balance
- Assess gait with patient's eyes open and closed
- Observation of gait
- Testing for peripheral neuropathy
- Spasticity evaluation

Testing
- Analysis in Gait Laboratory
- Berg balance testing
- Timed Get Up and Go
- Six-Minute Walk Test
- Computerized posturography

Pitfalls
- Not typically formally tested.

Red Flags
- Symptoms of hydrocephalus (NPH) or Parkinson disease

Treatment

Medical
- Treat spasticity if interfering with ambulatory ability

Exercises/rehabilitation
- Address components of gait (strength, coordination, sensory loss, special sensory dysfunction, pain)

- Gait training (best way to get someone to improve walking is to walk)
- Cardiovascular/aerobic training to optimize endurance.
- Strengthen core muscles of pelvis and distal musculature (gastrocnemius)
- Balance training
- Aquatic rehabilitation
- Body weight supported treadmill training
- Lower extremity bracing
- Functional electrical neuromuscular stimulation

Modalities
- Some evidence for vibratory platforms to enhance overall balance and mobility

Surgical
- None

Consults
- None

Complications/side effects
- Falls

Prognosis
- Majority (> 75%) will be able to ambulate in 5 months.
- If no improvement in ambulation by 3 months postinjury, small chance (< 15%) of ambulation recovery.

- Approximately 35% of patients with less than three-fifths lower extremity strength on manual muscle testing at rehabilitation admission require assistance with locomotion at discharge versus 11% of patients with three-fifths strength or better.

Helpful Hints
- Hip protectors have been demonstrated to significantly reduce injuries from falls; however, they must be worn at all times.
- Physical restraints have not been shown to reduce the risk of injury from falls; however, bed/chair alarms should be considered.
- Isolated lower extremity exercises are less effective at improving gait than repeated ambulation.

Suggested Reading
Katz D, White D, Alexander M, Klein R. Recovery of ambulation after traumatic brain injury. *Arch Phys Med Rehabil* 2004;85(6):865–869.

Section II: Conditions

Geriatric Traumatic Brain Injury

Description
- TBI accounts for 80,000 emergency visits per year for geriatric patients; 75% are admitted.
- Second highest incidence of TBI occurs in persons >65 years.
- Persons >75 years have highest overall mortality rate from TBI.
- Intracerebral lesions are 6 times more common than severe torso lesions in severe trauma in adults >70 years.

Etiology
- Causes include falls (51%), MVA (9%), assaults (1%), and unknown causes (21%).
- Suicide is third leading cause of injury-related mortality, behind falls and MVA.

Risk Factors
- Males have higher incidence.
- Females have higher rates of hospitalization.
- Fall risk factors include chronic sensory or muscular impairment, preexisting neurologic disorder, alcohol use, postural hypotension, medication effects, ill-fitting shoes or pants, environmental risks.
- Visual problems that impair driving

Clinical Features
- Older adults have more comorbidities than younger counterparts, in part due to premorbid medical problems (heart disease, diabetes, hypertension, coagulopathy due to warfarin use, dementia).
- Subdural hemorrhages are common due to the susceptibility of bridging vein shearing in the atrophied brain.
- The most common injuries include frontal lobe contusions, temporal lobe contusions, and subdural hematomas.
- Older adults may present later to emergency department/physician after fall, given natural progression of subdural hematoma (SDH).

Diagnosis

Differential diagnosis
- Elder abuse
- Stroke
- Normal pressure hydrocephalus
- Parkinson disease
- Delirium (medication, disease exacerbation, substance use)
- New onset or worsened dementia
- Stroke or TIA

History
- Standard TBI history

Exam
- Standard TBI examination

Testing
- Need to apply geriatric specific normal values for balance testing

Pitfalls
- With pseudomentia cerebri, depression may mimic dementia/delirium in older adults.

Red Flags
- Increasing rates of elder abuse have been associated with increasing TBI.

Treatment

Medical
- Primary focus of acute injury is to prevent/minimize secondary injury.
- Avoid narcotic medications if possible.
- Establish adequate nutrition.
- Consider timed voiding schedule if patient is incontinent after Foley catheter removal.
- Methylphenidate is first-line agent for hypoarousal.
- Selective serotonin agents are first-line for depression.
- For insomnia, low-dose trazadone or zolpidem are first-line options. Avoid benzodiazepines and tricyclic antidepressants.

Exercises
- Older adults at all age are able to tolerate and benefit from aerobic and anaerobic exercise.

- Alternative therapeutic environments (eg, day rehabilitation or skilled nursing facility) may be better suited to the slower pace often needed by older adults.

Modalities
- Standard modality interventions for symptoms

Surgical
- Neurosurgery

Consults
- Occupational therapy to assess
- Need for bathroom safety aides (tub benches, grab bars, etc)
- Need for long handled devices and reaches to accommodate for decreased flexibility
- Need for home evaluation to assess safety of house
- Geriatrics

Complications/side effects
- Premorbid conditions, including pain, arthritis, limited cardiopulmonary reserve, may limit rehabilitation efforts.

Prognosis
- Warfarin use associated with more severe TBI and higher mortality rates
- Dementia is associated with slower recovery from TBI.
- Elderly more likely to become physically and financially dependent on others after TBI

- Diffuse axonal injury associated with worse prognosis
- Very poor survival in individuals > 80 years old and with a Glasgow Coma Scale < 10.
- Individuals ≥55 years have longer lengths of stay in inpatient rehabilitation, slower recovery rates, and greater cognitive impairment at discharge compared to individual < 50 years when matched for injury severity.
- Old age is an independent predictor of worse outcome in TBI.

Helpful Hints
- Medicare Part A reimburses for acute care therapy, inpatient (IRF) and skilled (SNF) rehabilitation services, and durable medical equipment.
- Medicare Part B reimburses for physician visits, home health services, and outpatient and day therapy programs.
- Medicaid (varies by state) reimburses for inpatient and outpatient rehabilitation and custodial nursing home care.

Suggested Reading
Englander J, Cifu DX, Tran TT. The older adult. In: Zasler N, Katz D, Zafonte R, eds. *Brain Injury Medicine*. 1st ed. Demos; 2007:315–332.

Hearing Deficits

Description
- Sensory (sensorineural) hearing loss is due to dysfunction of the central auditory pathway.
- Conductive hearing loss is due to disorder in sound transmission.
- Sensorineural hearing loss is more common in TBI.

Etiology
- Vestibulocochlear (cranial nerve VIII) nerve injuries are commonly seen after temporal bone fractures.
- Temporal bone fractures can either be longitudinal or transverse.
- Transverse fractures have a 100% incidence of sensorineural hearing loss.
- Longitudinal fractures are associated more with conductive hearing loss (88%) or a mixed conductive/sensorineural hearing loss (12%).
- Longitudinal temporal bone fractures are associated with disruption in the ossicular chain anatomy and tympanic membrane tears.
- Disruption of the incudostapedial joint is the most common location of injury (82%).

Risk Factors
- Temporal bone fractures

Clinical Features
- Longitudinal bone fractures are correlated with hemorrhage from ear.

Diagnosis

Differential diagnosis
- Cerebellopontine tumors
- Spinocerebellar degeneration
- Impacted cerumen or foreign body
- Tympanic membrane tear
- Ossicular bone dislocations/fractures
- Presbycusis

History
- Vertigo
- Battle sign
- Mastoid fracture
- Hemorrhage from ear/otorrhea
- Vestibular complaints

Exam
- Ocular exam for nystagmus
- Otoscopic exam
- Audiology exam
- Posture testing (to assess vestibular portion of CN VIII)
- Dix-Hallpike maneuver—vestibular pathway injury
- Rinne test
  - Based on the principle that air conduction is better than bone conduction; however, when there is conductive hearing loss, bone can bypass the damaged conductive pathways.
  - A 512-Hz tuning fork is placed over mastoid process. Once sound is not audible, fork is placed over external auditory ear canal. If sound is still not audible, this implies conductive hearing loss.
- Weber test
  - Based on the principle that sound produced from a tuning fork placed on middle of forehead can be transmitted to the cochlea, thereby circumventing the middle ear.
  - Conductive hearing loss: ringing is louder on affected side.
  - Sensory hearing loss: ringing is less loud on affected side.

Testing
- Audiometrics (hearing test)
- Brainstem auditory evoked potentials in low level patients.

Pitfalls
- Clinical testing limited to patients with sufficient cognitive skills

Red Flags
- Variable or selective hearing deficits may be related to an acute intracerebral process (eg, hydrocephalus) or to psychological overlay.

Treatment

Medical
- Hearing aids
- Cochlear implants

Exercises/rehabilitation
- Adaptive strategies (visual scanning, alternative communication)

Modalities
- None

Surgical
- Surgical repair of ossicular bones

Consults
- Otolaryngology
- Audiology

Complications/side effects
- Individuals with persistent cognitive deficits may have difficulty adapting to the use of hearing aides or cochlear implants, despite the significant improvements in sound quality with current equipment and procedures.
- Tinnitus is a frequent side effect of an injury to the inner ear.

Prognosis
- Good prognosis for conductive hearing loss associated with temporal bone fracture (~80% recover).

Helpful Hints
- Horizontal nystagmus suggests peripheral lesion.
- Vertical nystagmus is always due to a central lesion.

Suggested Reading
Podoshin L, Fradis M. Hearing loss after traumatic brain injury. *Arch Otolaryngol* 1971;101:15–18.
Tos N. Prognosis of hearing loss in temporal bone fractures. *Laryngol Otol* 1971;85:1147–1159.

Section II: Conditions

Hemiparesis/Hemiplegia

Description
- Unilateral weakness typically contralateral to primary brain injury.
- Hemiparesis is weakness of a limb, whereas hemiplegia implies total absence of motor strength.

Etiology
- Most commonly seen with severe and focal TBI, rare with mild TBI (may occur transiently)
- Cerebral contusion
- Subdural or epidural hematoma

Risk Factors
- Focal brain injury

Clinical Features
- Unilateral weakness of arm and/or leg, usually more distal than proximal
- Sensory deficits are typically not dermatomal or neurotomal with TBI.
- Initially decreased tone that may progress to hypertonicity
- Initially decreased reflexes that may progress to hyperreflexia/clonus
- Hemiparetic upper extremities are prone to subluxation of the shoulder due to weakness across the shoulder girdle.
- Hemiparetic extremities are prone to nonpitting, distal, dependent edema due to impaired venous and lymphatic return caused by weakened muscle contraction.
- Hemiparetic lower extremities result in a gait pattern that consists of hip hiking, circumduction at the hip, genu recurvatum and foot drop.

Diagnosis

Differential diagnosis
- Stroke/aneurysm/arteriovenous malformation
- Multiple sclerosis
- Brain tumor
- Post-seizure (Todd) paralysis
- Myelopathy, including traumatic spinal cord injury
- Brachial/lumbar plexopathy
- Peripheral nerve injury
- Psychosomatic disorder

History
- Identify prior extremity weakness

Exam
- Perform complete motor, sensory, tone, muscle bulk, and deep tendon reflex examination.
- Assess shoulder for subluxation and/or pain.
- Assess hand and foot for edema.

Testing
- Brain imaging to define etiology of brain injury (TBI vs. stroke vs other)
- Spine imaging if history consistent with spine trauma or motor/sensory examination localizes lower motor neuron disorder
- Electrophysiologic testing to clarify differential diagnosis, eg, EEG for Todd paralysis, electromyogram for lower motor neuron disorder

Pitfalls
- Sensory deficits or neglect (inattention) may mimic or exacerbate weakness.
- Increased tone or spasticity may limit ability to determine degree of weakness.
- Weakened extremity may appear poorly coordinated despite intact cerebellum.
- Altered cognition may limit accuracy of evaluation.

Red Flags
- Increasing or variable weakness
- Dermatomal or neurotomal sensory deficits
- Nonanatomic weakness
- Extremity edema may be seen with hemiparesis; however, it may also be due to deep venous thrombosis, heterotopic ossification, or venous/lymphatic insufficiency.

Treatment

Medical
- None; no proven impact of medications

Exercises/rehabilitation

- Progressive, strengthening (resistive) exercises
- Patterned movements to restore function and enhance coordination
- Assistive and adaptive devices for persistent weakness
- Neuromuscular electrical stimulation for acute and chronic weakness
- Orthotic devices for persistent weakness
- Constraint-induced movement therapy for upper extremity is highly effective.
- Forced-use movement therapy, including body weight supported treadmill training for lower extremity
- Sensorimotor techniques to facilitate improved neurologic recovery and normal neurologic patterning, including those proposed by Bobath or Brunnstrom

Modalities

- Functional (neuromuscular) electric stimulation has been advocated for significant weakness. May be used as a substitute for weak muscles, but unclear it if enhances long-term recovery. Technical and cost limitations prevent wide-scale and regular usage.

Surgical

- Transplantation or transposition of alternative (unaffected) muscles for weak muscles may be considered; however, long-term results are limited and often poor. Significant motor relearning is necessary with all tendon/muscle transplantation; however, this presents an even greater challenge in individuals with persistent brain-injury–related cognitive and motor deficits.

Consults

- None

Complications/side effects

- Overuse injuries from repetitive exercise/activity can occur in the affected muscles and in the unaffected muscles that may be used to compensate for the weakness.
- Skin breakdown from orthotic devices
- Pain from neuromuscular electrical stimulation use.
- Shoulder subluxation may be seen with acute weakness across shoulder girdle.
- Shoulder adhesive capsulitis ("frozen shoulder") may be seen with weakness-related prolonged immobility.

Prognosis

- Hemiparesis affects approximately 30% of hospitalized patients with TBI acutely but only 3% at 4 months postinjury.
- Majority of recovery occurs within first 2 months of injury.
- Rate of recovery negatively correlated with initial weakness.
- Rate of recovery negatively correlated with overall injury severity.

Helpful Hints

- Persistent weakness 6 months postinjury is unlikely to improve spontaneously, and therapy is unlikely to be effective long-term unless limb can be used functionally on a daily basis.

Suggested Reading

Platz1 T, Hessel S, Mauritz K-H. Motor rehabilitation after traumatic brain injury and stroke: Advances in assessment and therapy. *Restor Neurol Neurosci* 1999;14(2–3):161–166.

Heterotopic Ossification

Description
- Lamellar bone formations in extraskeletal tissue
- 20% risk after moderate to severe TBI
- Most commonly involves the following joints (in decreasing order of involvement)—hips, elbows, shoulders, knees.
- Symptoms can begin as early as 2 weeks after inciting event.
- Can lead to nerve entrapment and joint ankylosis

Etiology
- Differentiation of osteoprogenitor stem cells in soft tissue as a result of an unknown process

Risk Factors
- Severe TBI
- Immobilization
- Duration of coma
- Spasticity
- Fractures, especially if open reduction internal fixation performed or in presence of joint dislocation

Clinical Features
- Limited range of motion across joint
- Localized inflammatory response
- Palpable mass
- Pain at area of inflammation

Diagnosis

Differential diagnosis
- Dependent edema
- Deep venous thrombosis
- Occult fracture
- Varicose veins
- Superficial thrombophlebitis
- Achilles tendonitis
- Ruptured Baker cyst
- Cellulitis
- Lymphedema
- Arterial insufficiency
- Hematoma

History
- Prior history of heterotopic ossification (HO)

Exam
- Full joint exam, including range of motion

Testing
- Creatine kinase—elevated in HO but nonspecific
- C-reactive protein elevated during inflammatory phase
- Serum alkaline phosphatase has little clinical value.

Imaging
- Triple phase bone scan using technetium-99 disphosphanate (TC-99) is gold standard.
  - TC-99 pools in areas of active bone activity
- Typically positive 2 weeks prior to radiographic evidence of HO
- In very early HO, only first pass flow or blood pool images may be abnormal (denoting hypervascularity of HO).
- Soft tissue uptake during the third phase is diagnostic of HO.
- Test lacks specificity for HO.
- Ultrasonography can detect HO at hips.
- Radiography lacks sensitivity in early HO when soft tissue calcification has not occurred.
- Approximately 7–10 days after clinical symptoms, signs of HO may be apparent on radiographs.

Pitfalls
- Diagnosis challenging in cognitively impaired or agitated patients.

Red Flags
- HO can lead to the development of pressure sores, deep venous thrombosis, vascular compression, or nerve compression.

Treatment

Medical
- Regular, controlled range of motion (oftentimes with premedication with pain medications)
- Indomethacin prophylaxis has been used in total hip arthroplasty 75 mg/day for 3 weeks.
- Radiation therapy has been used for both prophylaxis and/or treatment in total hip arthroplasty.

■ Bisphosphanates inhibit calcium-phosphate precipitation, slow hydroxyapatite crystal formation, and inhibit calcium-phosphate transformation to hydroxyapatite.

■ Inhibits bone crystallization not bone matrix formation

■ Must be continued for at least 6 months

■ 20 mg/kg/day orally for 3 months followed by 10 mg/kg/day orally for 3–6 months

■ Contraindicated in hypocalcemia and renal impairment

■ Use with caution if long bone fracture is present—may deter healing

Exercises

■ Regular, controlled passive ROM to prevent joint contracture

Modalities

■ Serial casting may be used to prevent acute joint contractures or to gradually reduce existing joint contractures; work by low intensity, long duration stretch.

Surgical

■ HO must reach maturity prior to resection (approximately 12–18 months)

■ Hemorrhage is most common complication.

Consults

■ Orthopedic surgery, if necessary

Complications/side effects

■ Nonsteroidal anti-inflammatory drugs like indomethacin affect the gastric, hepatic, and renal systems.

■ Bisphosphanates have mild gastrointestinal side effects, such as nausea and diarrhea.

■ Operative removal of HO carries a high morbidity with bleeding, infection, reankylosis, and HO recurrence being the most common complications.

Prognosis

■ HO has been associated with worse functional outcomes.

■ Early intervention has greatest impact.

Helpful Hints

■ Without daily aggressive ROM, patients will progressively lose ROM and usage of joint. Premedication with effective agents (narcotics) may be needed to facilitate activity.

Suggested Reading

Johns JS, Cifu DX, Keyser-Marcus L, Jolles PR, Fratkin MJ. Impact of heterotopic ossification on functional outcome after traumatic brain injury: A prospective analysis. *J Head Trauma Rehabil* 1999;14(3):269–276.

Varghese G. Heterotopic ossification. In: Berrol S, ed. Physical medicine and rehabilitation clinics of North America. Philadelphia, PA: Saunders; 1992;(3):407–415.

Section II: Conditions

Hyperesthesia

Description
- Hyperesthesia is a condition that involves an abnormal increase in sensitivity to stimuli of the senses, affecting tactile or special senses (auditory, gustatory, olfactory, or visual). Term predominantly used for tactile dysfunction

Etiology
- Injuries to the ventral posterolateral and ventral posteromedial nucleus of the thalamus may (rarely) result in hyperesthesia/pain

Risk Factors
- None

Clinical Features
- Increased, often painful, sensation to stimuli affecting limbs

Diagnosis

Differential diagnosis
- Peripheral nerve disorders
- Plexopathy
- Myelopathy
- Complex regional pain syndrome
- Chronic pain syndrome

History
- History of pain/hyperesthesia
- History of diabetes mellitus or alcohol abuse

Exam
- Pain score/diagram
- Two-point discrimination
- Stereognosis
- Light touch sensation
- Pin prick sensation
- Vibratory testing

Testing
- None

Red Flags
- Involvement of arm and leg on opposite sides is atypical of TBI.

Treatment

Medical
- Peripheral pain
  - Counterirritant liniments
- Central pain
  - Tricyclic antidepressants
  - Anticonvulsants
  - Methadone

Exercises/rehabilitation
- Desensitization techniques
- Pain management techniques

Modalities
- Peripheral and/or central nervous system electric stimulation (eg, transcutaneous electrical nerve stimulator or spinal cord stimulator)

Surgical
- None

Consults
- Otolaryngology for hyperacussis

Complications/side effects
- None

Prognosis

- No known role as prognostic indicator
- If symptoms are not improving by 3 months post-TBI, then unlikely to fully recover.

Helpful Hints

- No proven efficacy for narcotic pain medications.

Suggested Reading

Walker WC. Pain pathoetiology after TBI: Neural and nonneural mechanisms. *J Head Trauma Rehabil* 2004;19(1):72–81.

Hypoarousal

Description
- Decreased readiness to process environmental stimuli and/or information
- Commonly seen in individuals with severe TBI
- In less involved individuals may manifest with decreased alertness, inability to pay attention, or reduced mental speed

Etiology
- Malfunction of the reticulothalamic, thalamocortical, and/or reticulothalamic nervous system
- Bilateral injuries to the thalamus may cause a persistent vegetative or minimally conscious state.

Risk Factors
- Diffuse axonal injury
- Brain stem hemorrhage

Clinical Features
- Decreased alertness

Diagnosis

Differential diagnosis
- Medication effect
- Hypoxia
- Endocrinologic disturbance
  - Hypothyroidism
  - Hypoadrenalism
- Electrolyte disturbance
  - Hypoglycemia
- Hypomagnesia
  - Hypercalcemia
  - Hypophosphatemia
- Anemia
- Chronic infection
- Depression
- Hydrocephalus
- Acute neurologic insult (stroke, herniation syndrome, seizure)

History
- History of learning disability, including attention deficit/hyperactivity disorder

Exam
- Response to stimuli

Testing
- Thyroid function panel
- morning (AM) cortisol or cosyntropin stimulation test, if suspicious for hypoadrenalism
- Complete blood count
- Complete electrolyte panel including serum glucose, magnesium, and phosphorous
- Pulse oxygen testing

Pitfalls
- Diurnal variation in arousal is common.

Red Flags
- Change in pupillary response may indicate intracranial process.
- Change in neurologic status (hemineglect)

Treatment

Medical
- Methylphenidate
- Potentiates effects of dopamine and norepinephrine
- Half life 1.5–2.5 hours
- Side effects include insomnia, decreased appetite, abdominal discomfort, headaches, dizziness, motor tics
- May improve the rate of recovery, but not the final level of recovery
- Bromocriptine
- Agonist to dopamine type 2 receptor
- Treatment starts 2.5 mg/day and titrated up
- Side effects include dizziness, syncope, nausea, vomiting, abdominal cramping.
- Contraindicated in uncontrolled hypertension
- Main indicators for treatment are akinetic mutism, minimally conscious state

- Amantadine
- Potentiates dopamine; also uncompetitive antagonist of NMDA receptor
- Improves motivation, attention, alertness
- May improve abulia, mutism, perseveration
- Start at 50 mg twice daily
- Maximum dose 400 mg daily
- Side effects: headaches, nausea, orthostatic hypotension, anorexia, dizziness (anticholinergic type symptoms)
- May lower seizure threshold
- Modafinil
  - Unclear mechanism of action
  - May lower cortical GABA levels
- Start at 100 mg in am. Can be increased to 400 mg/day either in once-daily dosing or divided at am and noon.
- Carbidopa/L-Dopa
  - Less commonly used
  - No randomized controlled trials
- Start with low doses 10 mg/100 mg twice daily, and may be gradually increased to 25/250 mg four times daily
- Side effects include dyskinesias, anxiety, hallucinations, paranoia
- Amitriptyline
- Only case reports demonstrating improved arousal

Modalities
- None

Surgical
- None

Consults
- None

Complications/side effects
- Stimulant medications can cause insomnia if administered too late in the day.

Prognosis
- Poor after the acute period of injury (4 weeks)

Helpful Hints
- Enhancing environmental factors and stimuli will have as much effect as medications.

Suggested Reading
Whyte J, Polansky M, Fleming M, Coslett HB, Cavallucci C. Sustained arousal and attention after traumatic brain injury. *Neuropsychol* 1995;33(7):797–813.

Section II: Conditions

Hypoesthesia/Numbness

Description
- Hypoesthesia refers to a reduced sense of touch or sensation, or a partial loss of sensitivity to sensory stimuli.

Etiology
- The primary somatosensory cortex in the frontal lobe receives sensory stimuli from peripheral/afferent dorsal column neurons, medial lemniscal neurons, and thalamocortical neurons. Injuries to any of these structures can result in hypoesthesia.

Risk Factors
- None

Clinical Features
- Numbness

Diagnosis

Differential diagnosis
- Peripheral nerve disorders
- Plexopathy
- Myelopathy
- Tabes dorsalis (syphilis)

History
- History of numbness
- History of diabetes mellitus, alcohol abuse, thyroid disease, HIV, or syphilis

Exam
- Two-point discrimination
- Stereognosis
- Light touch sensation
- Pin prick sensation
- Vibratory testing

Testing
- Consider electrodiagnostic and evoked potentials testing

Pitfalls
- Perioral or tip of nose numbness are indicators of psychological overlay.

Red Flags
- Involvement of arm and leg on opposite sides is a typical of TBI.

Treatment

Medical
- None

Exercises/rehabilitation
- Enhanced awareness of affected areas to decrease risk of injury, such as frequent visual scanning

Modalities
- None

Surgical
- None

Consults
- None

Complications/side effects
- Elevated risk of burns (heating pad, hot pack) or skin irritation of affected area

Prognosis
- No known role as prognostic indicator
- If symptoms are not improving by 3 months post-TBI, then unlikely to recover.

Helpful Hints

- Home environment needs to be adjusted for safety concerns (eg, lower temperature of water heater).
- Daily visual skin inspection of affected areas

Suggested Reading

Cushman JG, Agarwal N, Fabian TC, et al. Practice Management Guidelines for the Management of Mild Traumatic Brain Injury: The EAST Practice Management Guidelines Work Group. *J Traum Inj Infect Crit Care*. 2001;51(5):1016–1026.

Hypotonia/Flaccidity

Description
- An upper or lower motor neuron abnormality resulting in decreased resting tension of muscle
- Hypotonia is a decrease in tone, whereas flaccidity is the total absence of tone.

Etiology
- Lower motor neuron lesion
- Acutely after upper motor neuron injury, a period (typically <2 weeks) of extremity hypotonia may be seen ("CNS shock").

Risk Factors
- Lower motor neuron injury

Clinical Features
- Decrease in muscle tension to passive range of motion
- Often accompanied by a decrease in motor stretch reflex across affected joints
- Hypotonia may affect oropharyngeal musculature, resulting in dysphagia and/or dysphonia.
- Muscle weakness is commonly associated with hypotonia.

Diagnosis

Differential diagnosis
- Traumatic injury to lower motor neuron (root or plexus)
- Nontraumatic lower motor neuron disease (poliomyelitis, infarction of limb with ischemic neuropathy)
- Concomitant spinal cord injury with acute spinal shock
- Post-seizure (Todd) paralysis
- Medication usage (benzodiazepine, dantrolene sulfate, lioresol)

History
- Identify prior history of hypotonia

Exam
- Perform complete motor, sensory, tone, and deep tendon reflex examination.
- Assess motor tone during passive and active range of motion.
- Evaluate for muscle atrophy and fasciculations.
- Assess swallowing and speech.

Testing
- Brain imaging to define etiology of injury (TBI vs CVA vs other).
- Spine imaging if history consistent with spine trauma or motor/sensory examination localizes lower motor neuron disorder
- Electrophysiologic testing to clarify differential diagnosis (EEG for Todd paralysis, EMG for lower motor neuron disorder)

Pitfalls
- Weakened extremity may appear poorly coordinated despite intact cerebellum.
- Tone may vary over the course of the day.

Red Flags
- Increasing hypotonia or weakness
- Nonanatomic weakness

Treatment

Medical
- None; no proven impact of medications

Exercises/rehabilitation
- Progressive, strengthening (resistive) exercises
- Patterned movements to restore function and enhance coordination
- Assistive and adaptive devices for persistent hypotonia with weakness
- Neuromuscular electrical stimulation for persistent hypotonia with weakness
- Orthotic devices for persistent hypotonia with weakness
- Constraint-induced movement therapy for upper extremity is highly effective for persistent hypotonia with weakness.
- Forced-use movement therapy, including body weight supported treadmill training for lower extremity
- Sensorimotor techniques to facilitate improved neurologic recovery and normal neurologic patterning, including those proposed by Bobath or Brunnstrom

Modalities

- Functional (neuromuscular) electric stimulation has been advocated for significant weakness, but unclear role with hypotonia. May be used as a substitute for weakened muscles, but unclear it if enhances long-term recovery. Technical and cost limitations prevent wide-scale and regular usage.

Surgical

- Transplantation or transposition of alternative (unaffected) muscles for weak muscles may be considered; however, long-term results are limited and often poor. Significant motor relearning is necessary with all tendon/muscle transplantation; however, this presents an even greater challenge in individuals with persistent brain-injury–related cognitive and motor deficits.

Consults

- None

Complications/side effects

- Overuse injuries from repetitive exercise/activity can occur in the affected muscles and in the unaffected muscles that may be used to compensate for the weakness.
- Skin breakdown from orthotic devices

- Pain from neuromuscular electrical stimulation use
- Shoulder subluxation may be seen with acute weakness across shoulder girdle.
- Shoulder adhesive capsulitis ("frozen shoulder") may be seen with weakness–related prolonged immobility.

Prognosis

- Majority of recovery occurs within first 6 months of injury.
- Rate of recovery negatively correlated with initial flaccidity.
- Rate of recovery negatively correlated with overall injury severity.

Helpful Hints

- Dantrolene sulfate can cause significant "hypotonia" (weakness) with overuse.
- Focal hypotonia is a common sign of a concomitant lower motor neuron injury after TBI.

Suggested Reading

Dieli J. Review of traumatic brain injury with orthotic considerations. *J Prosthet Orthot* 2002;14(1):31–35.

Insomnia

Description
- Insomnia is the most common sleep disorder after TBI.
- Disturbances in sleep after TBI may also be due to secondary disorders of obstructive sleep apnea (OSA), central sleep apnea (CSA), posttraumatic hypersomnia, periodic limb movements in sleep (PLMS), or restless leg syndrome (RLS), and narcolepsy.

Etiology
- Insomnia may be multifactorial, including sleep hygiene, medication, psychological, pain, and intrinsic brain injury issues.
- OSA is caused by the collapse of the pharynx against the glottis, which is normally held open by muscle activity.

Risk Factors
- Difficulties with psychomotor vigilance
- OSA: higher body mass index, neck circumference > 43 cm in men and > 37 cm in women, enlarged tonsils, high-arched palate, micrognathia

Clinical Features
- Patients may complain of difficulty in initiating or in maintaining sleep.
- Excessive daytime sleepiness
- OSA is characterized by snoring, witnessed apneic episodes, choking, sleep restlessness, morning headaches, daytime fatigue, and problems with memory or concentration.
- In narcolepsy, in addition to sleep attacks, cataplexy, sleep paralysis, and hypnogogic hallucinations may be seen.

Diagnosis

Differential diagnosis
- Depression
- OSA refers to cessation of breathing during sleep with the continued effort of breathing.
- CSA refers to the cessation of breathing with no neurologic effort to breath.
- Narcolepsy is a disorder of REM sleep that is characterized by fast REM onset and sleep attacks.
- PLMS is characterized by repeated rhythmic jerking of the extremities, usually the legs.

History
- Premorbid sleep disturbance
- Review of sleep hygiene (bedtime routine, stimulant ingestion, daytime napping)
- Physical activity log
- Medication review

Exam
- Inspect throat and oral cavity for potential obstructions

Testing
- Polysomnography is a sleep laboratory tool that measures breathing, respiratory muscle effort, muscle tone, and the divisions of sleep.
- Multiple Sleep Latency Test
- Gold standard objective assessment of sleepiness
- Measures time to fall asleep for 4–5 daytime naps
- Epworth Sleepiness Scale
- Self-administered questionnaire assessing likelihood of falling asleep during different situations

Pitfalls
- A number of medications for TBI care (anticonvulsants, antispasticity agents, pain agents) are sedating and may alter sleep–wake cycles.
- Daytime naps and resting may alter sleep–wake cycles.

Red Flags
- Morning headaches may be a sign of sleep apnea with morning hypercarbia.

Treatment

Medical
- Sleep hygiene

- Limit daytime sleeping to scheduled naps of decreasing duration and frequency, as wakefulness improves.
- OSA may benefit from continuous positive airway pressure.
- Hypersomnia
  - Stimulants (eg, methylphenidate)
- Narcolepsy
  - Stimulants (eg, methylphenidate)
- Clomipramine or fluoxetine for cataplexy
- Insomnia
  - Sleep hygiene
  - Sleep-inducing medications

Exercises
- Regular exercise program (not to be done in evening)

Modalities
- Sleep diary

Surgical
- OSA may benefit from urgical correction of upper airway including uvulopalatopharyngoplasty.

Consults
- Sleep disorder specialist
- Otolaryngologist

Complications/side effects
- Persistent sleepiness may impair ability to safely drive or operate machinery.

Prognosis
- Severe OSA is associated with increased cardiovascular mortality.

Helpful Hints
- OSA is a risk factor for hypertension, increased glucose levels, and glucose intolerance.

Suggested Reading
Thaxton LL, Patel AR. Sleep disturbances: Epidemiology, assessment and treatment. In: Zasler ND, Katz DI, Zafonte RD, eds. *Brain Injury Medicine.* New York: Demos; 2007:557–575.

Section II: Conditions

Locked-in Syndrome

Description
- Classic locked-in syndrome (LIS) includes complete quadriplegia, lower cranial nerve paralysis, and mutism, with preservation of consciousness, upper gaze, and upper eyelid movement.
- Incomplete or partial deficits related to pontine injury are often incorrectly labeled with LIS.

Etiology
- Insult to ventral pons due to trauma, tumor, hypotension, abscess, or ischemia (basilar artery obstruction via thrombus or air embolus)
- Rarely due to extensive damage of bilateral corticospinal and corticobulbar tracts
- Central pontine myelinolysis due to overly rapid correction of hyponatremia

Risk Factors
- Pontine lesion

Clinical Features
- No gender differences in etiology
- May see pseudobulbar affect with emotional lability (laughing, crying)
- Usually cognitively intact
- Can be classified into three categories
  - Total—total immobility (including paralyzed vertical eye gaze) and inability to communicate, with preserved consciousness
  - Classical—paralyzed vertical eye gaze, quadriplegia and anarthria with preserved consciousness and vertical eye movement. Head and facial movements are partially preserved.
  - Incomplete—paralyzed vertical eye gaze, quadriparesis, dysarthria, with preserved consciousness
- Most frequent causes of death are pulmonary complication and brainstem lesion extension.

Diagnosis

Differential diagnosis
- Akinetic mutism
- Vegetative state
- Subclinical seizures

History
- H/o CVA, transient ischemic attack, or seizures

Exam
- Standard TBI examination
- Observe for vertical gaze and voluntary blinking

Testing
- Magnetic resonance imaging to evaluate brainstem pathology

Pitfalls
- Concomitant cognitive deficits may initially limit communication attempts.

Red Flags
- Variable abilities to communicate may indicate more significant TBI, delirium, or psychological overlay.

Treatment

Medical
- Cognitive behavioral therapy for pseudobulbar lability
- Technical aides for communication

Exercises
- Daily range of motion exercises
- Focused exercises for muscles of > 3/5 strength

Modalities
- None

Surgical
- None

Consults
- Neurology

Complications/side effects
- Prone to complications of bed-bound patients (skin ulcers, contractures, deep venous thrombosis)

Prognosis

- As high as 80% 10-year survival reported, with greater survival if rehabilitation within 1 month
- Majority of individuals will have significant neurologic and functional deficits at 5 years.
- Motor recovery occurs in a distal to proximal pattern.
- Better prognosis for motor recovery if horizontal gaze intact
- Better prognosis seen in patients with vascular etiology

Helpful Hints

- Family usually first to note that patient is aware

Suggested Reading

Patterson JR, Grabois M. Locked-in syndrome: A review of 139 cases. *Stroke* 1986;17:758–764.

Minimally Conscious State

Description
- State of altered consciousness with minimal awareness of self and environment.
- Awareness can be occasional and inconsistent.
- Ranchos Los Amigos Cognitive and Behavioral Level III

Etiology
- Diffuse axonal injury
- Multifocal cortical contusions
- Less involvement of cortico-thalamic connections compared to vegetative state

Risk Factors
- Severe brain injury

Clinical Features
- Simple command following
- Intelligible verbalization
- Yes/no responses either verbal or with gestures (can be inaccurate)
- Recovery from minimally conscious state marked by functional object use

Diagnosis

Differential diagnosis
- Coma
- Vegetative state
- Locked-in syndrome
- Subclinical seizures

History
- Obtain observations by family, friends, therapists, and nurses regarding any purposeful behavior.

Exam
- Optimize patient-related factors for arousal.
- Minimalize environmental distractions and provide adequate lighting.
- Use simple language.
- Choose simple commands that patient will be able to perform within their motor capacity.
- Avoid asking patient to squeeze hand or blink eyes, as these can be reflexic actions.
- Purposeful movements include tracking or reaching for object in visual field.
- Look for purposeful behavior.
  - Try placing object in patient's hand, and see if they manipulate it.
  - Smiling or crying at picture of family member
  - Bringing toothbrush to mouth
  - Bringing hairbrush to hair
- Assess integrity of CNS.
- Brainstem evaluation includes pupillary reflexes, ocular movements, oculovestibular reflexes, gag reflex.
- May need serial assessment, as patient may be inconsistent.
- Standardized rating scales: JFK Coma Recovery Scale, Coma-Near Coma Scale

Testing
- Evoked potentials (somatosensory evoked potentials [SSEP], visual evoked potentials [VEP], brainstem auditory evoked potentials [BAEP]) and functional imaging (MRI, PET) may assist in differentiating coma vs near coma states, especially early in course of injury.
- The Coma–Near Coma Scale is a good monitoring tool that can be performed by a variety of clinicians.

Pitfalls
- Encephalomalacia on brain imaging is common after severe TBI with minimally conscious state and may be misinterpreted as hydrocephalus.

Red Flags
- Subtle declines in arousal level may indicate medical complication (eg, urinary tract infection); however, they may be hard to determine without uniform measurement system in place.

Treatment

Medical
- Sensory stimulation to improve arousal level
- Maintain ROM

- Management of common comorbidities (spasticity, heterotopic ossification, pressure ulcer, joint flexibility)
- Amantadine is first-line agent, but limited research support
- Bromocriptine: case reports demonstrate recovery of speech.

Exercises
- None

Modalities
- Median nerve (noxious) stimulation advocated but limited scientific support

Surgical
- Deep brain stimulation, but limited scientific support

Consults
- Neurology, if suspect seizure activity limiting arousal
- Neurosurgery, if suspect hydrocephalus limiting arousal

Complications/side effects
- Amantadine lowers the seizure threshold and should be used with care.

Prognosis
- Compared to vegetative state, patients in a minimally conscious state demonstrate a longer period of recovery and less functional disability at 12 months.
- Mortality rates similar to those of vegetative state
- Better prognosis for those with traumatic vs nontraumatic injury

- If unconscious at 1 month, 33% will regain consciousness by 3 months postinjury, 46% by 6 months, and 53% by 1 year.
- If unconscious at 3 months, only 35% chance of recovery by 1 year.
- If unconscious at 6 months postinjury, only 16% chance of consciousness at 1 year.
- Prognosis for consciousness very poor if consciousness not present by 1 year postinjury
- 50% of patients will be severely disabled and 33% moderately disabled by 12 months postinjury.
- If > 40 years, worse functional outcome
- Mortality rates are higher for patients that have been in a minimally conscious state for at least 1 month.
  - 82% mortality at 3 years
  - 95% mortality at 5 years.

Helpful Hints
- There may be significant variability in the level of arousal throughout the day related to fluctuating cognitive function or sleep–wake cycling.
- Consistent monitoring of cognitive/arousal status using standardized scales (CNC, JFK Coma Recovery Scale) is recommended to uniformly assess status.
- Significant (consistent) worsening on standardized scales may indicate evidence medical decline (eg, urinary tract infection) rather than an acute cerebral process.

Suggested Reading
Giacino J, Ashwal S, Childs N, et al. The minimally conscious state: Definition and diagnostic criteria. *Neurol* 2002;58:349–353.

Neglect (Unilateral Spatial Inattention)

Description
- Visual-perceptual disorders include unilateral spatial inattention (neglect), cortical blindness, impaired color perception, visual agnosia, visual-spatial disorders, and visual-constructive disorders.
- Pure unilateral spatial inattention occurs when an individual involuntarily fails to respond to stimuli on one side despite having intact sensory and motor systems.
- Patients may deny they have a problem (anosognosia) or fail to express any emotional response to their impairments (anosodiaphoria).
- Unilateral spatial inattention is frequently accompanied by visual field cuts, paresis, and decreased tactile and stereognostic perception of the involved side. The intact hemisphere remains oblivious to the deficits of the involved hemisphere.

Etiology
- Non-dominant inferior parietal lobe lesions are most common, but also seen in lesions of the dorsolateral frontal lobe, thalamus, and putamen.

Risk Factors
- Nondominant hemisphere trauma

Clinical Features
- Orientation of activities predominantly toward the attended space
- Head, trunk, eyes rotated toward side of lesion
- Scanning of eyes only in attended space (despite full extraocular movements)
- Eating only half a plate of food
- Reading only half a page
- Bumping into doorways on unattended side
- Veering toward the attended space when trying to follow a straight line

Diagnosis

Differential diagnosis
- Hemianopia
- Conversion disorder
- Migraine
- Other brain injury

History
- Prior vision status, including diplopia, field cuts

Exam
- Double simultaneous stimulation testing to evaluate for extinction
- Line bisection tasks: individual is asked to bisect line on a piece of paper placed at midline.
- Drawing tasks: individual is asked to draw a clock or a flower.

Testing
- Optokinetic nystagmus testing

Pitfalls
- Extinction cannot be tested if patient unable to detect a single stimulus on one side of the body.

Red Flags
- Worsening signs of neglect may indicate either an acute intracranial abnormality or worsening behavioral difficulties.

Treatment

Medical
- Minimal evidence of efficacy; however, dopaminergic drugs may be useful.

Exercises
- Visual scanning (lighthouse method)—eye movements without head movements are major goal.
- Progressive transference of tasks from attended spaces to unattended spaces during therapy (including therapist position next to the patient).
- Computer-assisted therapy

Modalities
- Visual (lights) and auditory (bells) stimuli on extremities may improve attention.

Surgical

■ None

Consults

■ Visual rehabilitation specialist
■ Neuro-ophthalmology if concomitant visual field cut

Complications/side effects

■ Elevated risk for self-injury related to decreased awareness of the body in the environment (eg, bumping into things)

Prognosis

■ Initial deficits are associated with worse functional outcomes and longer acute hospital stays

■ Persistent deficits at 3 months are indicative of poor long-term recovery and of overall poor prognosis.
■ In individuals with neglect, concomitant anosognosia has a poorer prognosis for functional recovery.

Helpful Hints

■ Individuals with pure hemianopsia are aware of the visual loss and will compensate by moving their eyes toward the lost visual field (in contrast to unilateral spatial inattention).

Suggested Reading

Pavlovskaya M, Ring H, Groswasser Z, Hochstein S. Searching with unilateral neglect. *J Cognit Neurosci* 2002;14(5);745–756.

Neuroendocrine Dysfunction: Other

Description
- Central diabetes insipidus (DI) results in hypernatremia from a decreased secretion of antidiuretic hormone.
- Growth hormone (GH) deficiency results from a decreased secretion of growth hormone.
- Hypothyroidism results from a decrease in thyroid-stimulating hormone (TSH).
- Hyperprolactinemia results from a decrease in cerebral dopamine that causes an increase in prolactin release (ie, prolatin is under tonic inhibition if dopamine).
- Adrenal insufficiency results from a lack of corticotrophin-releasing hormone or corticotropic hormone.
- Precocious puberty results from an increase in circulating gonadotropin-releasing hormone (GnRH).

Etiology
- Trauma to or hemorrhage to the pituitary gland resulting from injury in the midbrain and brainstem

Risk Factors
- Moderate to severe TBI
- DI: facial and basilar skull fractures

Clinical Features
- DI presents with polydipsia and polyuria, but patient may be clinically normal if adequate water is available for hydration.
- GH deficiency presents with fatigue, a decrease in muscle mass, exercise intolerance, truncal obesity, and confusion.
- Hypothyroidism presents with typical features, including constipation, fatigue, cold intolerance, dry skin, peripheral edema, hair loss, and late effects hyporeflexia with delayed muscle relaxation and bradycardia.
- Hyperprolactinemia presents with galactorrhea, menstruation abnormalities, hypogonadism, sexual dysfunction, and visual field deficits.
- Adrenal insufficiency presents with weakness, fatigue, weight loss, hypoglycemia, postural hypotension, anorexia, and abdominal pain.
- Precocious puberty presents, in children, with early development of pubic hair and breasts (in girls).

Diagnosis

Differential diagnosis
- Other causes of endocrine dysfunction

History
- Prior symptoms of endocrine dysfunction

Exam
- General systemic examination
- General neurologic examination
- Cognitive examination

Testing
- DI: urine specific gravity > 1.005, urine osmolarity < 200, plasma osmolarity > 200
- DI: water deprivation test, for chronic mild abnormality, will result will unmask condition.
- GH deficiency: rule out hypothyroidism, IGF-1 and IGFBP-3 low
- GH deficiency: positive response to insulin injection
- Hypothyroidism: TSH low, free T4 low
- Hyperprolactinemia: rule out hypothyroidism, prolactin levels high
- Adrenal insufficiency: am cortisol levels low, serum aldosterone low, cosyntropin stimulation test positive
- Precocious puberty: sex hormones high

Pitfalls
- Hyperprolactinemia: evaluate for medications that deplete dopamine (methyldopa) or are dopamine antagonists (metoclopramide, risperidone).

Red Flags
- N/A

Treatment

Medical
- DI: demopressin (DDAVP) nasal spray; vasopressin
- GH deficiency: somatotropin
- Hypothyroidism: levothyroxine
- Hyperprolactinemia: correct hypothyroidism; bromocriptine mesylate
- Adrenal insufficiency: if aldosterone deficient, give fluodrocortisone, hydrocortisone, dexamethasone, prednisone
- Precocious puberty: GnRH analogue; GnRH agonist

Exercises
- N/A

Modalities
- N/A

Surgical
- N/A

Consults
- Endocrinology

Complications/side effects
- N/A

Prognosis
- Most patients will resolve by 3 months after injury; however, if persistent after, then it is unlikely to ever resolve.

Helpful Hints
- DI usually presents 10 days after injury.
- GH: GH therapy has been associated with increased intracranial pressure.
- Hypothyroidism: in patients with cardiac disease, administer small amounts of levothyroxine and titrate up slowly.
- Hyperprolactinemia: rule out pregnancy as cause.
- Adrenal insufficiency: too much glucocortioid replacement will lead to Cushing Syndrome.

Suggested Reading

Barreca T, Perria C, Sannia A, et al. Evaluation of anterior pituitary function in patients with posttraumatic diabetes insipidus. *J Clin Endocrinol Metab* 1980;51(6):1279–1282.

Section II: Conditions

Neuroendocrine Dysfunction: Syndrome of Inappropriate Antidiuretic Hormone

Description
- Syndrome characterized by excessive release of antidiuretic hormone (ADH or vasopressin) from the posterior pituitary gland or another source
- The result is hyponatremia, and sometimes fluid overload.
- Most common endocrinologic cause of hyponatremia (low serum sodium) after brain injury

Etiology
- Excessive release of antidiuretic hormone from the posterior pituitary gland or another source due to intracranial injury to the midbrain and brainstem.

Risk Factors
- Prior h/o syndrome of inappropriate antidiuretic hormone (SIADH)

Clinical Features
- Often asymptomatic unless serum sodium is < 125 but may present with worsening arousal or cognition.
- If untreated, seizures can result.

Diagnosis

Differential diagnosis
- Central salt wasting
- Nephropathy
- Psychogenic water intoxication
- Thiazide diuretic use

History
- Prior h/o SIADH

Exam
- Cognitive status evaluation

Testing
- Urine and serum osmolality

Pitfalls
- Risk of dehydration and renal failure with fluid restriction

Red Flags
- Seizures

Treatment

Medical
- Fluid restriction (1200–1500 mL/day)
- Furosemide with replacement of sodium and potassium
- Demeclocycline

Exercises
- N/A

Modalities
- N/A

Surgical
- N/A

Consults
- Endocrinology

Complications/side effects
- Seizures may arise from hyponatremia (usually below 120).

■ Avoid demeclocycline in hepatic failure.

Prognosis
■ Excellent with rapid treatment of hyponatremia
■ Most patients respond rapidly to fluid restriction.

Helpful Hints
■ Should see improvements in sodium within 48 hours of fluid restriction (1200 mL/day)

Suggested Reading
Stewart DG, Cifu DX. Management of neuroendocrine disorders after brain injury. *Phys Med Rehabil Clin N Am* 1997;8(4):827–842.

Neurolinguistic Deficits of Traumatic Brain Injury

Description
- Pragmatic (use of language in context) deficits associated with diffuse brain injury
- May not be detected by traditional language assessment tools and aphasia screening batteries

Etiology
- Diffuse axonal damage that involves the organization of semantic information

Risk Factors
- Frontal lobe injury

Clinical Features
- Reduction in number of different words produced
- Greater frequency of verbal paraphasias
- Increased incidence of grammatical errors (word order transpositions, verb tense errors)
- Impaired planning and organization of language (decreased ability to convey multiple ideas into single sentences)
- Decreased meaningful conceptual links between sentences
- Decreased quality of information (redundant, off-topic information)
- May see more word retrieval and syntax impairments earlier on after injury
- Impaired story generation
- Impaired participation in conversation, especially if unfamiliar with conversant
- Impairments in recognition of emotion
- Impairments in interpretation of sarcasm

Diagnosis

Differential diagnosis
- Aphasia due to focal lesion
- Premorbid language deficits

History
- Premorbid language deficits

Exam
- Analysis of narrative, conversational discourse

Testing
- Microlinguistic and macrolinguistic analysis
- Wisconsin Card Sorting Test for measures of story narratives
- Test of Language Competence
- Neurosensory Centre Comprehensive Examination for Aphasia
- Boston Naming Test
- Wiig-Semel Test of Linguistic Concepts
- Boston Diagnostic Aphasia Examination

Pitfalls
- Pragmatic assessments do not take into consideration the social roles an individual with TBI would like to fulfill.

Red Flags
- Worsening language deficits

Treatment

Medical
- Limited efficacy with medications; however, acetylcholinesterase inhibitors, methylphenidate, and amantadine may be considered

Exercises
- Behavioral approaches may be more appropriate if individual has little insight into deficits (rewarding short answers with social praise in an individual with circumlocutory speech).
- Practice personally relevant communication task.
- Videotaping sessions to evaluate performance

Modalities
- None

Surgical
- None

Consults
- Speech language pathology, in particular, specializing in discourse analysis

Complications/side effects
- None

Prognosis
- Commonly seen after TBI with good resolution in most, related to severity
- Poor prognosis if little or slow recovery by 6 months

- Younger age at time of injury (< 5 years old) has poorer prognosis for linguistic recovery

Helpful Hints
- The "confused language" of brain injury does not easily fit into commonly used aphasia classification systems for stroke patients.

Suggested Reading
Coehlo CA, Liles BZ, Duffy RJ. Impairments of discourse abilities and executive functions in traumatically brain injured adults. *Brain Inj* 1995;9(5):471–477.

Pain: Complex Regional Pain Syndrome

Description
- Term for pain syndrome involving the upper or lower extremity that persists despite management of all acute factors
- Unclear if complex regional pain syndrome (CRPS) is an actual physiologic phenomenon or merely a label for a myriad of chronic pain conditions
- Most commonly affects proximal (hip, shoulder) and distal (foot, hand) aspects of extremity and not mid-section (knee, elbow)
- May involve nocioceptive, neuropathic, or inflammatory components
- As with all pain syndromes, psychologic factors play a significant role.

Etiology
- Unclear; previously felt to be related to autonomic dysfunction

Risk Factors
- Prior pain conditions
- Diabetes mellitus
- Hyperthyroidism
- Burns
- Myocardial infarction
- Entrapment neuropathies
- Fractures in affected limb

Clinical Features
- Divided into three stages
  - Acute stage: involves burning or aching in limb, edema, and faster rate of hair or nail growth.
  - Dystrophic stage (3–6 months after injury): edema, burning pain, hypothermia, increased muscle tone
  - Atrophic phase (6 months after injury): painful movement, contractures, temperature intolerance, subcutaneous tissue atrophy

Diagnosis

Differential diagnosis
- Postphlebitic syndrome
- Dependent edema
- Adhesive capsulitis
- Spasticity
- Entrapment neuropathies
- Peripheral neuropathy

History
- Prior painful conditions or syndromes

Exam
- Evaluate for swelling, allodynia, hair/nail changes, limitation of movement

Testing
- Three-phase bone imaging may aid in diagnosis.
- Consider specialized autonomic testing (diagnostic sympathetic blocks).

Pitfalls
- Postphlebitic syndrome has many of the same features as CRPS and occurs in one-third of untreated extremity DVTs.

Red Flags
- Symptom magnification and secondary gain issues play a role in many chronic pain conditions.

Treatment

Medical
- Advise smoking cessation
- NSAIDs for early pain relief
- Capsaicin cream for mild symptoms
- Low-dose amitriptyline
- Gabapentin and pregabulin have been advocated for neuropathic symptoms
- Oral corticosteroids may be considered in severe cases
- Sympathetic nerve blocks

Exercises
- Structured aerobic exercise has been demonstrated to decrease the perception of pain.
- Regular and progressive joint flexibility and range of motion are important to prevent contractures and functional limitations form pain syndromes.

Modalities
- Transcutaneous electrical nerve stimulation
- Progressive desensitization

Surgical
- Surgical sympathectomy for refractory cases

Consults
- Pain management

Complications/side effects

■ Chronic pain syndrome with associated functional limitations

Prognosis

■ As with any pain syndrome, persistence of symptoms past 6 months is associated with poorer long-term outcome.

Helpful Hints

■ The duration of stages is variable among patients

Suggested Reading

Harden N. Pharmacotherapy of complex regional pain syndrome. *Arch Phys Med Rehabil* 2005;84(S3):17–28.

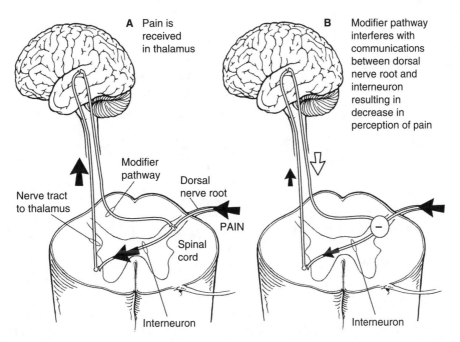

Proposed pathways for acute pain transmission. (With permission from Zasler ND, Katz DI, Zafonte RD. *Brain Injury Medicine: Principles and Practice.* New York: Demos Medical Publishing; 2007.)

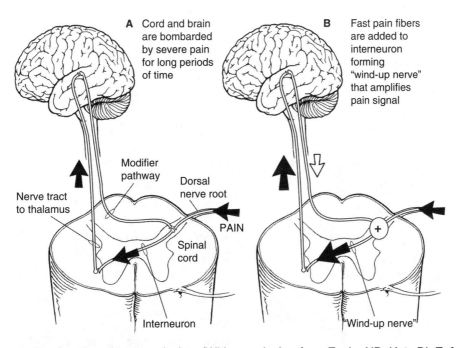

Proposed pathways for chronic pain transmission. (With permission from Zasler ND, Katz DI, Zafonte RD. *Brain Injury Medicine: Principles and Practice.* New York: Demos Medical Publishing; 2007.)

Pain: General

Description
- Physiological pain is the unpleasant awareness of a noxious stimulus or bodily harm. In pathologic pain, the unpleasant sensation is present in the absence of these stimuli or in the presence of nonnoxious stimuli.
- Pain is influenced by medical, cultural, societal, and psychological factors.

Etiology
- TBI with polytrauma may be accompanied by acute nociceptive (physiologic) pain from posttraumatic headaches, fractures, abrasions, wounds, burns, spasticity, deep venous thrombosis, heterotopic ossification, IVs/tracheostomies/gastrostomy tubes, constipation, urinary retention, and other noxious stimuli.
- Central (neuropathic) pain is typically diffuse pain attributed to central nervous system damage, primarily in the thalamus (see Hyperesthesia, page 100)

Risk Factors
- Polytrauma
- Headaches associated with cervical injuries and more commonly reported in mild TBI

Clinical Features
- In the minimally conscious patient, may see increased agitation with pain
- Central pain may be diffuse pain or may also be seen as hyperesthesia, allodynia, and/or dysesthesias involving half of the body.
- See Pain: Headaches, page 126.

Diagnosis

Differential diagnosis
- Neuropathic pain from peripheral nerve injuries structures
- Physiologic pain from secondary medical conditions (Heterotopic Ossification (HO), DVT, fracture)
- Degenerative or mechanical spinal pain
- Chronic regional pain syndrome (CRPS)
- Fibromyalgia

History
- History of pain conditions
- Pain coping strategies
- Depression screen

Exam
- Perform complete cranial nerve, motor, sensory, tone, and deep tendon reflex examination.
- Pain assessment scale
- Screen for undiagnosed fractures.
- Screen for deep venous thrombosis.
- Screen for range of motion on heterotopic ossification.
- Evaluation of allodynia, hyperalgesia, dysesthesias
- Evaluate for urinary retention/fecal compaction.
- Evaluate temporal mandibular joint in patients with posttraumatic headache.
- Evaluate for spasticity.
- In cognitively or communication-impaired patients, look for increased tone/posturing, tachycardia, tachypnea.

Testing
- Electromyogram/Nerve conduction study for peripheral nerve lesions/radiculopathy
- Consider triple phase bone scan for heterotopic ossification or CRPS.
- Consider duplex Doppler ultrasound of affected limb to evaluate for DVT.

Pitfalls
- Patients with altered awareness may make diagnosis difficult or misleading.
- Undertreatment of pain in patients with altered consciousness is common.
- Sedating pain mediations may limit cognitive function and recovery.

Red Flags
- Worsening behavioral dysfunction may be caused by undertreated pain.

Treatment

Medical
- Encourage and promote sleep hygiene.

- Nociceptive pain
  - For acute mild pain, acetaminophen and NSAIDs
  - For acute moderate pain, NSAIDs and tramadol
  - For acute severe pain, opioids
  - Consider adjuvant analgesics for moderate or severe pain.
    ○ Antidepressants
    ○ Anticonvulsants
- Central pain
  - Tricyclic antidepressants
  - Anticonvulsants
  - Methadone
- Posttraumatic headaches: See Pain: Headaches
- CRPS: role for select SSRI and neuropathic medications, along with sleep normalization and psychological counseling
- Spasticity: See Spasticity/Hypertonicity/Rigidity/Clonus

Exercises
- Relaxation techniques
- Biofeedback
- Encourage home exercise program

Modalities
- Superficial heat/cold
- Transcutaneous electrical nerve stimulation units
- Traction for cervical pain (in cognitively intact patients only)

Surgical
- Deep brain stimulators for central pain

Consults
- None

Complications/side effects
- Use caution with tramadol as it can lower the seizure threshold.

Prognosis
- No known role as prognostic indicator
- If symptoms are not improving by 3 months post-TBI, unlikely to fully recover

Helpful Hints
- Avoid narcotics if possible as they dull cognition and have addictive properties.
- Beware of burns in minimally conscious patients when using thermal modalities.

Suggested Reading
Zasler ND, Horn LJ, Martelli MF, Nicholson K. Post-traumatic pain disorders: Medical assessment and management. In: Zasler ND, Katz DI, Zafonte RD, eds. *Brain Injury Medicine*. New York: Demos; 2007:697–721.

Section II: Conditions

Pain: Headaches

Description
- Common complaint after head injury, most common after mild TBI

Etiology
- Sources of pain include
  - Dura
  - Venous sinuses
  - Cranial cavities (sinuses, ears, nasal cavities, orbits)
  - Cervical/cranial joint capsules
  - Cervical sympathetic plexus
  - Cervical myofascial tissue

Risk Factors
- Whiplash injury

Clinical Features

Subtypes of headache
- Musculoskeletal headache
  - Caplike discomfort
  - Relieved by application of heat, cold, or massage
- Cervicogenic headache
  - Dysfunction of facet joints
  - Unilateral head pain usually suboccipital
  - C2 and C3 facet dysfunction radiates to the head
- Neuritic head pain
  - May be due to local blunt trauma, penetrating injury, or surgical excision
  - Patient may report numbness or dysesthesias
- Neuralgic head pain
  - Nerves involved include occipital, supraorbital, infraorbital, and facial
  - Stabbing pain
- Posttraumatic migraine
  - Throbbing, unilateral, exacerbated by coughing
  - May present with nausea and vomiting
- Posttraumatic tension headaches
  - Tension headache is most common nontraumatic cause for headaches.
  - Characterized by bilateral, viselike discomfort

Diagnosis

Differential diagnosis
- Analgesic rebound headache
- Trigeminal neuralgia
- Temporal mandibular joint (TMJ) symptoms
- Late intracranial hemorrhage
- Tension pneumocephalus due to dural leaks
- Hydrocephalus
- Ventriculoperitoneal shunt failure
- Posttraumatic epilepsy

History
- Premorbid history of headaches
- Mechanism of head injury
- Assess for acceleration/deceleration forces at injury
- H/o neurosurgical intervention
- Complete description of pain: character, onset, location, duration, exacerbating factors, relieving factors, severity, frequency
- Assess for associated symptoms (photophobia, aura, nausea, vomiting)

Exam
- Neurologic exam
- Cervical range of motion
- Palpation of cranial/cervical musculature
- Palpation of temporomandibular joints
- Provocative maneuvers of cervical spine (Spurling maneuver, distraction test, compression test)

Testing
- Cervical spine imaging

Pitfalls
- Mixed etiology of symptoms is common.

Red Flags
- Acute or worsening neurologic symptoms are indicative of intracranial pathology.

Treatment

Medical
- Musculoskeletal or tension headaches
  - Nonsteroidal anti-inflammatory medications (NSAIDs)
  - Tricyclic antidepressants (TCAs)
  - Neurolytic (eg, botulinum toxin) injections
  - If craniomandibular disorder, try softer food consistency and jaw exercises.
- Cervicogenic headache
  - Local anesthetic injection intra-articularly

– Medial branch block of the dorsal rami
– Osteopathic techniques
■ Neuritic/neuropathic pain
– NSAIDS
– TCAs
– Anticonvulsants (eg, gabapentin, pregabalin)
– Duloxetine
■ Posttraumatic migraine
– Prophylaxis includes NSAIDS, β-blockers, calcium channel blockers, TCAs, and depakote.
– Abortive medication, include dihydroergotamine derivatives, triptans, narcotics.
– Neurolytic (eg, botulinum toxin) injections

Exercises
■ Biofeedback muscle relaxation exercises
■ Musculoskeletal flexibility and posture

Modalities
■ Transcutaneous electrical nerve stimulation (TENS)
■ Desensitization techniques

Surgical
■ Rarely surgical decompression or nerve lysis is needed for neuropathic pain.

Consults
■ Neurology
■ Pain management

Complications/side effects
■ Side effects from the multiple pain medications commonly used, including polypharmacy, are common.

Prognosis
■ More than 95% of posttraumatic headaches will resolve within 4 weeks.
■ Late developing (> 2 weeks postinjury) may not be related to actual TBI.

Helpful Hints
■ Headaches are more common after mild TBI and with cranial surgery.

Suggested Reading
Lew HL, Lin P-H, Fuh J-L, Wang S-J, Clark DJ, Walker WC. Characteristics and treatment of headache after traumatic brain injury: A focused review. *Am J Phys Med Rehabil* 2006;85:619–627.

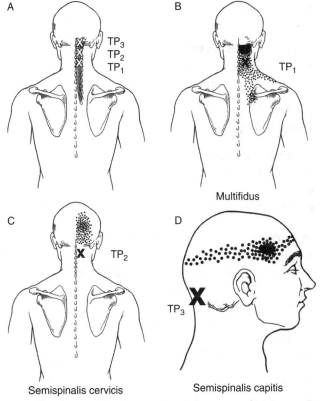

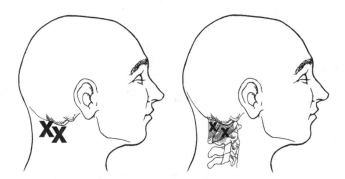

Suboccipital muscle trigger points. (With permission from Zasler ND, Katz DI, Zafonte RD. *Brain Injury Medicine: Principles and Practice.* New York: Demos Medical Publishing; 2007.)

Posterior cervical muscles prone to development of trigger points producing referred pain perceived as cervicalgia and/or cephalalgia. (With permission from Zasler ND, Katz DI, Zafonte RD. *Brain Injury Medicine: Principles and Practice.* New York: Demos Medical Publishing; 2007.)

Pediatric Traumatic Brain Injury

Description
- Leading cause of acquired disability in children

Etiology
- Common causes are motor vehicle accidents, falls, sports and recreational activities, child abuse, and assault
- Majority of children < 15 years involved in motor vehicle collisions are pedestrians or bicyclists.

Risk Factors
- H/o child abuse or neglect
- Male gender

Clinical Features
- Typical features of TBI
- Higher rate of early posttraumatic seizures

Diagnosis

Differential diagnosis
- Acute chemical poisoning
- Chronic lead poisoning
- Alcohol or drug use

History
- H/o child abuse
- H/o alcohol or drug use must be considered.

Exam
- Complete neurologic examination, tailored to pediatric population
- See Shaken Baby Syndrome

Testing
- No pediatric specific testing needed; follow recommendations based on presentation

Pitfalls
- Limited functional assessment possible in young children.

Red Flags
- Child abuse must be considered with pediatric TBI.

Treatment

Medical
- Standard medication interventions for symptoms

Exercises
- Standard rehabilitation interventions for symptoms

Modalities
- Standard modality interventions for symptoms

Surgical
- Pediatric neurosurgery

Consults
- Return-to-school activities occur during acute rehabilitation.
- Community reintegration services
  - Child may require special education services.
  - An individual education plan (IEP) can be formulated that allows for modifications to assist with cognitive or physical deficits.
  - IEP should be reviewed frequently as improvements in function can still occur after TBI.
- Social worker
- Teacher

Complications/side effects
- Similar to adult TBI

Prognosis
- Psychosocial outcomes linked more closely to preinjury family function than injury severity
- For mild TBI, children may have headaches and subtle cognitive deficits.
  - May want to ease back into school with half days

- For severe TBI, prognosis is better than adults, but most patients fail to show complete recovery.
- 75% of children will regain consciousness after having been unconscious for greater than 90 days.
- Worse outcomes associated with children who have been abused
- Limited research specifically addressing prognosis in children/teens compared with adults

Helpful Hints
- Seat belt laws have significantly lowered the frequency and severity of pediatric TBI.

- Bicycle helmet clearly helps prevent TBI.
- Encourage use of helmets with bike riding.
- Encourage proper restraints to be used in vehicles.
- Lower rates of deep venous thrombosis than adults
- Precocious puberty may be a sign of neuroendocrine dysfunction.

Suggested Reading
Sumich AI, Nelson MR, McDeavitt JT. TBI: Pediatric perspective. In: Zasler ND, Katz DI, Zafonte RD, eds. *Brain Injury Medicine.* New York: Demos, 2007, 305–313.

Section II: Conditions

Penetrating Injuries

Description
- Projectile passes through cranium and brain, resulting in brain injury.

Etiology
- Primary injury
  - Trauma due to the impact of the projectile
  - Bullets damage brain tissue via crushing, cavitation, and shock waves.
  - In stab wounds, cerebral damage is usually restricted to wound tract.
- Secondary injury
  - Pathologic processes that occur due to the primary injury and deter recovery

Risk Factors
- Violence-related TBI
- Combat-related TBI

Clinical Features
- Victims of gunshot wounds to the head are 35 times more likely to die than victims of similar nonpenetrating brain injuries.
- Bullet impact can cause cavitation 3–30 times larger than the size of the bullet.
- Stab wounds usually occur through thin bones of the skull, notably the orbital surfaces and squamous portion of the temporal bone.

Diagnosis

Differential diagnosis
- None

History
- Standard TBI history

Exam
- Standard TBI exam

Testing
- Computerized tomography (CT) scan of head

Pitfalls
- Higher incidence of late effects of injury, especially hydrocephalus, intracranial infection, and posttraumatic seizures.

Red Flags
- Retained skull fragments can be a source of infection that can manifest with worsening or variable arousal or cognition.
- Often need craniectomy after penetrating injury

Treatment

Medical
- Seizure prophylaxis for 1 week postinjury

Exercises
- No specific modifications or precautions related to injury
- Protective helmet needed with craniectomy

Modalities
- None

Surgical
- Typically requires surgical debridement initially
- Cranioplasty after craniectomy may be performed by 6 weeks postsurgery.

Consults
- Neurosurgery
- Trauma surgery
- Skull prosthetist

Complications/side effects
- At risk for the following medical complications
  - Intracranial infections, including posttraumatic meningitis, cranial epidural abscess, subdural empyema, and brain abscesses
  - Posttraumatic epilepsy rates are 2 times that of nonpenetrating TBI
  - Posttraumatic cerebrospinal fluid leak
  - Cranial nerve injuries, especially facial nerve injury, if temporal bone fractured

– Pseudoaneurysm
– Arteriovenous fistulas
– Hydrocephalus, related to intracranial bleeding

Prognosis

- Lower mortality rates seen in stab wounds with penetrating object initially left in place (11%) vs removed (26%)
- Worse outcome associated with high intracranial pressures and hypotension
- CT findings associated with worse outcome include
  – Bihemispheric injury
  – Intraventricular hemorrhage
  – Subarachnoid hemorrhage
  – Midline shift
  – Uncal herniation
- Mortality rates are as high as 90% for those patients with penetrating brain injury and postresuscitative GCS of 3–5.

- More favorable prognosis seen in victims of gunshot wounds with Glasgow Coma Score (GCS) > 8

Helpful Hints

- Patients with penetrating injury require closer short- and long-term monitoring, given the higher incidence of secondary complications.

Suggested Reading

Black KL, Hanks RA, Zafonte RD, et al. Blunt versus penetrating violent brain injury: Frequency and factors associated with secondary conditions and complications. *J Head Trauma Rehabil* 2002;17(6):489–496.

Grahm TW, Williams FC, Harrington T, et al. Civilian gunshot wounds to the head: A prospective study. *Neurosurg* 1990;27(5):696–700.

Section II: Conditions

Posttraumatic Amnesia

Description
- Time from injury to return of continuous memory and orientation
- Type of delirium unique to traumatic brain injury (TBI)

Etiology
- Any TBI that results in persistent altered consciousness

Risk Factors
- Moderate to severe TBI

Clinical Features
- Usually significantly longer than retrograde amnesia
- Unlike retrograde amnesia, there is no preferential sparing of the oldest memories once PTA resolves.
- Rarely uniform in severity across all areas of cognition
- Patients can demonstrate learning through interventions that demonstrate consistency and repetition; new information acquisition is less impaired than recall of that new information.

Diagnosis

Differential diagnosis
- Altered mental status due to metabolic abnormality
- Medications that cause sedation
- Alcohol/illicit drugs

History
- Often estimated retrospectively
- Galveston Orientation and Amnesia Test (GOAT) is the most commonly used test to measure PTA
  - Score of 75 or more (range from 0–100) on three consecutive occasions at least 8 hours apart is considered to indicate that patient is out of posttraumatic amnesia (PTA).
  - Research validated for all severities of TBI

Exam
- Assessment of attention, concentration, orientation, and memory

Testing
- Galveston Orientation and Amnesia Test (GOAT)
- Orientation Group Monitoring System (OGM)
- Westmead PTA Scale

Pitfalls
- Medical conditions that prevent assessment (intubations, severe pain, sedating medications)
- Medical conditions that exacerbate or cause cognitive difficulties (seizures, infection, metabolic abnormalities, hypoxia, or pain)
- Sleep deprivation may exacerbate thinking difficulties.

Red Flags
- Worsening level or consciousness or orientation is indicative of acute process other than TBI.

Treatment

Medical
- Stabilize medical condition
- Discontinue sedating medications if possible
- Allow alcohol/drugs to clear system

Exercises/rehabilitation
- Appropriate environmental stimulation
- Memory log/assistance

Modalities
- Personal digital assistant (PDA) and programmed pagers can provide structured cueing.

Surgical
- None

Consults
- Psychology, neuropsychology, speech and language pathology, occupational therapy

Complications/side effects

Prognosis
- Duration of PTA can help determine prognosis in TBI.
  - Predictive of functional outcome, return to work, occurrence of posttraumatic epilepsy, degree of cognitive recovery
- Resolution of PTA often correlates with when a patient benefits most from a comprehensive rehabilitation program.
  - Less agitation
  - Better attention span
  - Better tolerance for activity

- Older age is associated with a lesser chance of clearing PTA

Helpful Hints
- Modified GOAT available for patients with aphasia
- Pediatric version (COAT) available

Suggested Reading
Amed S, Bigsley R, Sheikh JI, Date ES. Post-traumatic amnesia after closed head injury: A review of the literature and some suggestions for future research. *Brain Inj* 2000;14:765–780.

Posttraumatic Hydrocephalus

Description
- Increase in volume or pressure of cerebrospinal fluid (CSF) in the central nervous system
- Two major types: communicating and noncommunicating
  - In communicating hydrocephalus, there is full continuity between ventricles and subarachnoid space.
  - In noncommunicating hydrocephalus, there is blockage of flow in the ventricular system or outlet to the subarachnoid space.
- May present with increased (acute presentation) or normal (subacute or chronic presentation) intracranial pressure

Etiology
- Communicating
  - Overproduction of CSF (choroid plexus tumor)
  - Insufficient absorption of CSF at arachnoid granulations
  - Is usually caused by impaired absorption at the arachnoid villi, presumably due to blood (ie, subarachnoid hemorrhage) or inflammatory mediators (meningitis)
- Noncommunicating
  - Blockage of CSF flow by hematoma or mass

Risk Factors
- Increased age
- Intracranial infection
- Intracranial hemorrhage
- Intracranial fragments

Clinical Features
- Failure to improve during acute period after TBI or later neurologic/functional decline
- Headaches
- Frontal release signs
- Bulging craniectomy flap
- Vomiting
- Blurred vision, related to papilledema
- Urinary incontinence
- Double vision, most commonly due to cranial nerve VI palsy
- Drowsiness
- If normal pressure hydrocephalus, may see classic triad of gait disorder, urinary incontinence, and memory impairment

- In acute hydrocephalus, may see Cushing's triad of hypertension, bradycardia, and hypoventilation

Diagnosis

Differential diagnosis
- Cerebral atrophy (ie, hydrocephalus ex vacuo)
- Any loss of cerebral tissue leading to compensatory ventricular enlargement
- Congenital hydrocephalus

History
- History of symptom duration and rapidity, timing, and nature of head trauma

Exam
- Ophthalmoloscopic exam
- Extraocular movements, to assess failure of upward gaze or cranial nerve VI palsy
- Gait evaluation
- Frontal release signs

Testing
- CT
- Magnetic resonance imaging of ventricular system is neuroimage of choice.
- CSF tap test
  - Lumbar puncture to assess for CSF pressure (normal 110 mm water)
  - Observe for improvement in cognitive and functional status after removing 50 mL of CSF

Pitfalls
- Imaging of the brain should precede CSF tap test as herniation risk is increased in patients with severely elevated ICP.
- Patients with severe TBI often develop encephalomalacia 1–6 months postinjury: may be confused with focal hydrocephalus on brain imaging.

Red Flags
- Cerebral herniation

Treatment

Medical
- Occasionally used as temporizing measure before surgery

■ Acetazolamide or furosemide decrease rate of CSF production

■ Isosorbide may increase rate of CSF absorption

Exercises
■ None

Modalities
■ None

Surgical
■ Placement of CSF shunt—ventriculoperitoneal, ventriculoatrial, or lumboperitoneal.

■ Ventricular shunt is usually right sided to avoid language centers of brain

■ Serial LPs can be done initially after intraventricular hemorrhage because hydrocephalus may be temporary

■ Other neurosurgical interventions include
  – Opening of stenosed aqueduct
  – Choroid plexectomy
  – Choroid plexus coagulation
  – Endoscopic fenestration of floor of third ventricle, which provides alternative route of flow for CSF

Consults
■ Neurosurgery
■ Ophthalmology

Complications/side effects
■ Shunt complications include infection, shunt failure, occlusion, overshunting, and placement errors.

Prognosis
■ Significant improvements usually seen within 3 months of shunting

■ In patients with communicating hydrocephalus after TBI, there are longer durations of coma and a greater severity of behavioral problems.

Helpful Hints
■ In addition to typical signs of confusion, incontinence, and imbalance, hydrocephalus may present with headache, hypertension, or bradycardia.

Suggested Reading
Mazzini L, Campini R, Angelino E, Rognone E, Pastore I, Oliveri G. Posttraumatic hydrocephalus: A clinical, neuroradiologic and neuropsychologic assessment of long-term outcome. *Arch Phys Med Rehabil* 2003;84:1637–1641.

Section II: Conditions

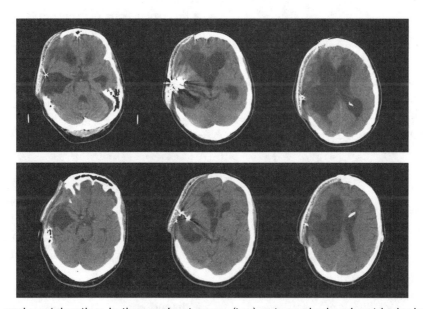

Hydrocephalus pre- and postshunting. In the preshunt scans (top) note marked periventricular lucency in the white matter consistent with transependymal fluid in addition to ventricular enlargement. There is also artifact from aneurysm clip and right hemispheric encephalomalacia, maximal in the right temporal lobe. Postshunt scans show persisting encephalomalacia of the right hemisphere including the right lateral ventricle and right temporal horn. Shunt is now seen entering the left lateral ventricle, which has now normalized (including left temporal horn), and periventricular lucency has largely resolved. (With permission from Zasler ND, Katz DI, Zafonte RD. *Brain Injury Medicine: Principles and Practice.* New York: Demos Medical Publishing; 2007.)

Posttraumatic Seizures

Description

- Definitions
  - Immediate posttraumatic seizures (PTS) occur within first 24 hours after traumatic brain injury (TBI).
  - Early PTS occur within first week after TBI.
  - Late PTS occur after first week of TBI.
  - Posttraumatic epilepsy is recurrent late PTS.
- Incidence
  - Occurs in 5% to 7% of hospitalized patients with TBI
  - Occurs in > 10% of severe nonpenetrating TBI victims
  - Occurs in 35% to 50% of patients with severe penetrating TBI

Etiology

- Not clearly understood

Risk Factors

- GCS < 10
- Depressed skull fracture
- Injuries with dural penetration
- Midline shift > 5 mm
- Multiple intracranial operations
- Intracerebral hemorrhage
- Cortical contusion
  - Biparietal contusion
- Epidural hematoma
- Subdural hematoma
- Seizure within first week of injury
- Prolonged length of coma
- Prolonged length of posttraumatic amnesia

Clinical Features

- Most common seizure type is complex partial seizure, followed by simple partial and then tonic-clonic (grand mal) seizures.
- Temporal lobe epilepsy may result in acute alterations in behavior (acute rage).

Diagnosis

Differential diagnosis

- Seizures due to metabolic abnormalities (hyper- or hypoglycemia, hyponatremia) or hypoxia

- Pseudoseizures
- Anoxic myoclonus
- Encephalomyelitis
- Meningitis
- Drug intoxication
- Drug withdrawal
- Tremors
- Febrile seizures (in children)

History

- Complete TBI exam
- Evaluate circumstances and characteristics of event
- Complete review of systems, especially constitutional symptoms of fevers, chills, neck rigidity
- Medication review
- Substance abuse history

Exam

- Complete TBI exam
- Assess for nuchal rigidity

Testing

- Electroencephalogram (EEG)
  - EEG findings do not show a direct association with increased risk of early or late PTS.
- Complete blood count, comprehensive metabolic panel including hepatic panel, magnesium, and phosphorus
- Urine toxicology screen
- Alcohol level
- Lumbar puncture if meningitis suspected

Pitfalls

- Simple partial seizures can involve special senses, ie, olfactory lobe with acute unpleasant smell, visual cortex with acute visual changes/hallucinations, parietal cortex with acute alterations in sensation, or auditory cortex with acute auditory changes/hallucinations.
- Temporal lobe (behavioral) epilepsy can be difficult to diagnose.

Red Flags

- Pseudo- or psychogenic seizures are more likely to manifest during periods of increased stress and are more likely to vary in clinical presentation.

Treatment

Medical

- There is no evidence that treating immediate, nonstatus epilepticus-type seizures reduces risk of developing early or late seizures.
- All individuals with acute moderate or severe TBI benefit from 7 days of phenytoin use to reduce the incidence of early PTS. Use of antiepileptic drug (AEDs) prophylaxis after TBI for more than 7 days does not lessen incidence of developing late PTS.
  - Effective for tonic-clonic and complex partial seizures
  - Available in parenteral form; however, the intravenous form (fosphenytoin) can lower mean arterial pressure, leading to cerebral hypoperfusion
- Early seizures should be treated for a minimum of 3 months, with many clinicians advocating for a treatment duration of 1 to –2 years.
- Discontinue medications that lower the seizure threshold (meperidine, tramadol, beta-lactam antibiotics, isoniazid, quinolones, cyclosporine, tacrolimus, theophylline)

Exercises

- None

Modalities

- Deep brain stimulation for temporal lobe epilepsy

Surgical

- Brain tissue resection by neurosurgery (ie, corpus callosotomy, temporal lobectomy)

Consults

- Neurology

Complications/side effects

- All AEDs have cognitive side effects, with phenobarbital having the greatest potential.
- AEDs may impede neurologic recovery.

Prognosis

- Early PTS are associated with increased risk of late PTS.
- 50% to –66% of individuals with late PTS will experience first seizure within 12 months.
- 75% of individuals with late PTS will experience first seizure within 24 months.

Helpful Hints

- Risk of epilepsy greatest during first 2 years after injury
- Most patients can be treated with monotherapy of AEDs.
- The incidence of PTS in patients receiving chronic AED therapy has been reported to be higher than those patients not receiving prophylaxis; however, this may be related to treater bias (treaters seem to know who is at higher risk of seizing, but medications may have limited effect).

Suggested Reading

Yablon SA, Dostrow VG. Post-traumatic seizures and epilepsy. In: Zasler ND, Katz DI, Zafonte RD, eds. *Brain Injury Medicine*. New York: Demos; 2007:443–468.

Section II: Conditions

Posttraumatic Stress Disorder

Description

- Posttraumatic stress disorder (PTSD) is an anxiety disorder that can develop after exposure to one or more traumatic events that threatened or caused great physical harm.
- May be seen in concert with TBI
- Can be present with TBI even if there is no active memory of injury (eg, with severe TBI).
- PTSD has also been recognized in the past as railway spine, stress syndrome, shell shock, battle fatigue, traumatic war neurosis, or posttraumatic stress syndrome.

Etiology

- It is a severe and ongoing emotional reaction to an extreme psychological trauma.

Risk Factors

- Although most people (50%–90%) encounter trauma over a lifetime, only about 8% develop full PTSD. Vulnerability to PTSD presumably stems from an interaction of biological diathesis, early childhood developmental experiences, and trauma severity.
- Traumatic events that may cause PTSD symptoms to develop include violent assault, kidnapping, sexual assault, torture, being a hostage, prisoner of war or concentration camp victim, experiencing a disaster, violent automobile accidents, or getting a diagnosis of a life-threatening illness.
- Witnessing traumatic experiences or learning about these experiences may also cause the development of PTSD symptoms.
- The amount of dissociation that follows directly after a trauma predicts PTSD: individuals who are more likely to dissociate during a traumatic event are considerably more likely to develop chronic PTSD.
- Members of the Marines and Army are much more likely to develop PTSD than Air Force and Navy personnel, because of greater exposure to combat.
- A preliminary study found that mutations in a stress-related gene interact with child abuse to increase the risk of PTSD in adults.

Clinical Features

- Symptoms include re-experience, such as flashbacks and nightmares; avoidance of stimuli associated with the trauma; and increased arousal, such as difficulty falling or staying asleep, anger, and hypervigilance.
- Individuals tend to avoid places, people, or other things that remind them of the event and are exquisitely sensitive to normal life experiences.
- Untreated PTSD can have devastating, far-reaching consequences for sufferers' functioning in relationships, their families, and in society.

Diagnosis

- The diagnostic criteria for PTSD, per *DSM-IV-TR*:
  A. Exposure to a traumatic event
  B. Persistent re-experience (eg, flashbacks, nightmares)
  C. Persistent avoidance of stimuli associated with the trauma (eg, inability to talk about things at all related to the experience, avoidance of things and discussions that trigger flashbacks, reluctance to re-experiencing symptoms, fear of losing control)
  D. Persistent symptoms of increased arousal (eg, difficulty falling or staying asleep, anger and hypervigilance)
  E. Duration of symptoms more than 1 month
  F. Significant impairment in social, occupational, or other important areas of functioning (eg, problems with work and relationships.)
- Criterion A (the "stressor") consists of two parts, both of which must apply for a diagnosis of PTSD. The first (A1) requires that "the person experienced, witnessed, or was confronted with an event or events that involved actual or threatened death or serious injury, or a threat to the physical integrity of self or others." The second (A2) requires that "the person's response involved intense fear, helplessness, or horror."

Differential diagnosis

- Acute stress reaction
- Depression
- Schizophrenia

- Psychosocial overlay related to malingering, secondary gain (benefits, service connectiveness)
- Alcohol/drug usage
- Postconcussive syndrome

History
- Exposure to event (trauma, near trauma, violence, sexual) that may have had severe psychological effect

Exam
- Standard general physical examination
- Standard TBI examination

Testing
- Individuals diagnosed with PTSD respond more strongly to a dexamethasone suppression test than individuals diagnosed with clinical depression.
- Most people with PTSD also show a low secretion of cortisol and high secretion of catecholamines in urine, with a norepinephrine/cortisol ratio consequently higher than comparable nondiagnosed individuals.
- Brain catecholamine levels are low, and corticotropin-releasing factor (CRF) concentrations are high.
- Neuroimaging may reveal a decrease in hippocampal volume.

Pitfalls
- Concurrent substance abuse is common.
- Concurrent TBI and/or pain syndrome may limit ability to identify single source of psychological distress.
- Limited research supporting the treatment of PTSD with concurrent TBI or pain syndrome

Red Flags
- Elevated suicide risk
- Symptoms may worsen during periods of substance abuse withdrawal.

Treatment

Medical
- Medications have shown benefit in reducing PTSD symptoms but rarely achieve complete remission. Standard medication therapy useful in treating PTSD includes SSRIs (selective serotonin reuptake inhibitors) and TCAs (tricyclic antidepressants).

Exercises
- General conditional and fitness recommendations

Modalities
- Relaxation strategies

Surgical
- None

Consults
- Many forms of psychotherapy have been advocated for trauma-related problems such as PTSD. Basic counseling for PTSD includes education about the condition and provision of safety and support.
- The psychotherapy programs with the strongest demonstrated efficacy include cognitive behavioral programs, variants of exposure therapy, stress inoculation training, variants of cognitive therapy, eye movement desensitization and reprocessing, and many combinations of these procedures.

Complications/side effects
- Antidepressant medication often reduce appetite, so close monitoring of oral intake is warranted for the first 2 to 4 weeks after beginning or increasing medication dosing.

Prognosis
- Good response is seen with early detection and intervention, primarily using psychological management.
- Unclear prognosis with concurrent conditions (eg, TBI, substance abuse, chronic pain)

Helpful Hints
- Interdisciplinary management is a key to management.

Suggested Reading
Kessler RC, Sonnega A, Bromet E, Hughes M, Neslon CB. Posttraumatic stress disorder in the National Comorbidity Survey. *Arch Gen Psychiatr* 1995;52:1048–1060.

Warden DL, Labbate LA, Salazar AM, et al. Posttraumatic stress disorder in patients with traumatic brain injury and amnesia for the event. *J Neuropsychiatry Clin Neurosci* 1997;9:18–22.

Section II: Conditions

Pressure Sores

Description
- Skin breakdown is influenced by many factors, such as unrelieved pressure, friction, humidity, shearing forces, temperature, age, incontinence, and medications affecting cognition.
- Skin breakdown can occur at any body part, but especially portions over bony or cartilaginous areas.
- Most commonly seen after TBI in individuals who are immobilized due to severe cognitive (eg, coma), physical (eg, spasticity), or behavioral (eg, pulling out indwelling tubes) deficits or who have behavioral deficits that result in self-injury

Etiology
- Unrelieved pressure, shearing forces, and irritation from incontinence are the most common causes after TBI.

Risk Factors
- Cognitive deficits (TBI-related, medication-related, preexisting)
- Behavioral deficits
- Sensory deficits
- Incontinence
- Quadriparesis
- Profound hypertonia or spasticity
- Older age
- Long-term local or systemic steroid usage

Clinical Features
- Pressure ulcers are commonly staged by severity:
  - Stage I is the most superficial, indicated by nonblanchable redness that does not subside after pressure is relieved.
  - Stage II is damage to the epidermis extending into, but no deeper than, the dermis. In this stage, the ulcer may be referred to as a blister or abrasion.
  - Stage III involves the full thickness of the skin and may extend into the subcutaneous tissue layer.
  - Stage IV is the deepest, extending into the muscle, tendon, or even bone.

Diagnosis

Differential diagnosis
- Hyperemia from pressure
- Burns
- Healed pressure sore with scarring
- Cellulitis
- Laceration from trauma

History
- H/o pressure ulcer
- H/o fragile skin (skin tears, discoloration)
- H/o long-term local or systemic steroid usage

Exam
- Standard general physical examination, with focus on integument
- Standard TBI examination

Testing
- Consider bone scan or CT scan for poorly healing stage III or IV pressure ulcers to assess for underlying abscess or osteomyelitis.
- Consider sterile bone biopsy to assess for osteomyelitis.

Pitfalls
- Wound or skin cultures are rarely diagnostic.

Red Flags
- Chronic osteomyelitis will prevent wound healing and is a common cause of breakdown of healed pressure ulcers.

Treatment

Medical
- Treatment of underlying infections
- Wound care products and dressings to maintain cleanliness of area, reduce bacterial overgrowth, enzymatic debridement of necrotic tissue, appropriate moisture balance to ulcer, and reduce the risk of local trauma.

Exercises/rehabilitation
- Reduction of pressure with frequent turning and off-loading of focal pressure points

Modalities

- Edema management

Surgical

- Prudent debridement of nonviable tissue

Consults

- Plastic surgery
- Wound care team

Complications/side effects

- Draining open wounds may contribute to low serum albumin.
- Significant source of delays in progression in rehabilitation programs.
- Chronic osteomyelitis may contribute to hemolysis and resultant anemia.

Prognosis

- Pressure ulcers that occur during the acute phase of injury will typically resolve rapidly when pressure is completely relieved from the area, unless underlying infection, poor nutrition, skin maceration from moisture or bodily fluids, or significant shear forces are present.
- Pressure ulcers that are chronic in nature or due to chronic deficits from injury (eg, spasticity, contracture) are more difficult to resolve

Helpful Hints

- In children, the disproportionately large size of the head will predispose them to occipital pressure ulcers when forced to spend time in bed or wheelchair (with a head support).
- While newer debridement agents and bio-occlusive dressings are extremely effective, removing pressure to the affected area is the predominant intervention required.

Suggested Reading

Dimant J. Implementing pressure ulcer prevention and treatment programs: Using AMDA clinical practice guidelines. *JAMDA* 2001;2:315–325.

Section II: Conditions

Stage I	Stage I	Stage III	Stage IV
Nonblanchable erythema of intact skin, the heralding lesion of skin ulceration. In individuals with darker skin, discoloration of the skin, warmth, edema, induration, or hardness may also be indicators.	Partial-thickness skin loss involving epidermis, dermis or both. The ulcer is superficial and presents clinically as an abrasion, blister, or shallow crater.	Full-thickness skin loss involving damage to or necrosis of subcutaneous tissue that may extend down to, but not through, underlying fascia. The ulcer presents clinically as a deep crater with or without undermining of adjacent tissue.	Full-thickness skin loss with extensive destruction, tissue necrosis, or damage to muscle, bone, or supporting structures (eg, tendon, joint capsule). Undermining and sinus tracts also may be associated with stage IV ulcers.
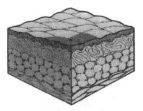	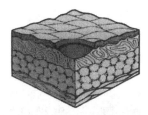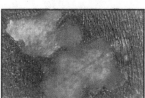	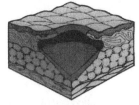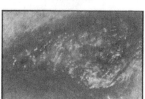	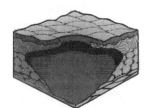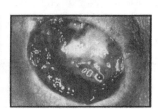

- Stage I ulcers may not always be diagnosed reliably in patients with darkly pigmented skin.
- When eschar is present, a pressure ulcer cannot be staged accurately until the eschar is removed.
- Be alert to pressure-induced pain in patients with casts or support stockings.

The National Pressure Ulcer Advisory Panel pressure ulcer staging system. (With permission from Zasler ND, Katz DI, Zafonte RD. *Brain Injury Medicine: Principles and Practice.* New York: Demos Medical Publishing; 2007.)

Quadriparesis

Description
- Weakness of all four extremities
- Quadriparesis is weakness of the extremities, whereas quadriplegia implies total absence of strength.

Etiology
- Severe TBI with bilateral involvement of motor cortex
- Brainstem TBI, especially pontine involvement

Risk Factors
- Multifocal TBI
- Brainstem injury

Clinical Features
- Quadriparesis/quadriplegia results in significant functional limitations, often necessitating total care (initially).
- Bowel and bladder continence are more often impaired than in focal weakness.
- Bilateral weakness of arm and/or leg, usually more distal than proximal
- Sensory deficits are typically not dermatomal or neurotomal with TBI.
- Initially decreased tone that may progress to hypertonicity
- Initially decreased reflexes that may progress to hyperreflexia/clonus
- Weak upper extremities are prone to subluxation of the shoulder due to weakness across the shoulder girdle.
- Weak extremities are prone to nonpitting, distal, dependent edema due to impaired venous and lymphatic return caused by weakened muscle contraction.
- Weak lower extremities result in a gait pattern that consists of hip hiking, circumduction at the hip, genu recurvatum, and foot drop.

Diagnosis

Differential diagnosis
- Coma/vegetative state
- Locked-in syndrome
- Myopathy
- Neuromuscular junction disorders
- Neuropathy, especially critical illness neuropathy
- Myelopathy, including traumatic spinal cord injury

History
- Identify prior extremity weakness.

Exam
- Perform complete motor, sensory, tone, and deep tendon reflex examination.
- Assess shoulders for subluxation and/or pain.
- Assess hands and feet for edema.

Testing
- Brain imaging to define etiology of brain injury (TBI vs CVA vs other)
- Spine imaging if history consistent with spine trauma or motor/sensory examination localizes lower motor neuron disorder.
- Electrophysiologic testing to clarify differential diagnosis, eg, EEG for Todd paralysis, EMG for lower motor neuron disorder

Pitfalls
- Sensory deficits or neglect (inattention) may mimic or exacerbate weakness.
- Increased tone or spasticity may limit ability to determine degree of weakness.
- Weakened extremity may appear poorly coordinated despite intact cerebellum.

Red Flags
- Increasing weakness
- Dermatomal or neurotomal sensory deficits
- Nonanatomic weakness
- Extremity edema may also be due to DVT, HO, or venous/lymphatic insufficiency

Treatment

Medical
- None

Exercises/rehabilitation
- Progressive, strengthening (resistive) exercises
- Patterned movements to restore function
- Assistive and adaptive devices for persistent weakness

- Neuromuscular electrical stimulation for acute and chronic weakness
- Orthotic devices for persistent weakness
- Constraint-induced movement therapy for upper extremity is highly effective.
- Forced use movement therapy, including body weight supported treadmill training for lower extremity
- Sensorimotor techniques to facilitate improved neurologic recovery and normal neurologic patterning, including those proposed by Bobath or Brunnstrom

Modalities

- Functional (neuromuscular) electric stimulation has been advocated for significant weakness. May be used as a substitute for weak muscles, but unclear if it enhances long-term recovery. Technical and cost limitations prevent wide-scale and regular usage.

Surgical

- Transplantation or transposition of alternative (unaffected) muscles for weak muscles may be considered; however; long-term results are limited and often poor. Significant motor relearning is necessary with all tendon/muscle transplantation; however, this presents an even greater challenge in individuals with persistent brain injury-related cognitive and motor deficits.

Consults

- None

Complications/side effects

- Overuse injuries from repetitive exercise/activity can occur in the affected muscles and in the unaffected muscles that may be used to compensate for the weakness.
- Skin breakdown from orthotic devices
- Pain from neuromuscular electrical stimulation use
- Shoulder subluxation may be seen with acute weakness across shoulder girdle
- Shoulder adhesive capsulitis ("frozen shoulder") may be seen with weakness-related prolonged immobility.

Prognosis

- Recovery anticipated to take longer than with focal weakness
- Majority of recovery occurs within first 6 months of injury.
- Rate of recovery negatively correlated with initial weakness.
- Rate of recovery negatively correlated with overall injury severity.

Helpful Hints

- Persistent weakness 6 months postinjury is unlikely to improve spontaneously, and therapy is unlikely to be effective long-term unless limb can be used functionally on a daily basis.

Suggested Reading

Kanyer B. Meeting the seating and mobility needs of the client with traumatic brain injury. *J Head Trauma Rehabil* 1992;7(3):81–93.

Spinal Cord and Traumatic Brain Injury: Dual Disability

Description
- More than 25% of patients with spinal cord injury (SCI) suffer brain injury, perhaps ≥60%
  - 11% of patients who suffer from SCI also have a severe TBI.
  - 50% sustain mild TBI.
- Motor vehicle accidents are more highly associated with severe TBI.

Etiology
- Similar to common causes of TBI

Risk Factors
- Male
- Alcohol use
- Participation in contact sports
- Motor vehicle collisions
- Level of spinal cord injury is positively correlated with risk of TBI, with C1–C4 level (regardless of completeness) having highest risk and T1-S3 (motor incomplete) the lowest.

Clinical Features
- Symptoms of mild TBI
- Central dysautonomia involves rigidity, fevers, tachycardia, sweating.

Diagnosis

Differential diagnosis
- Pre-existing cognitive deficits (TBI, dementia)
- Pre-existing behavioral disorder
- Depression

History
- Alteration or loss of consciousness at time of injury
- Amnesia for events at time of injury

Exam
- Standard TBI examination

Testing
- If milder injury, may not see any abnormalities on magnetic resonance imaging and computerized tomography scan.
- Formal neuropsychological testing

Pitfalls
- Missed diagnosis of TBI or SCI

Red Flags
- SCI deficits may appear worse initially than would be expected from injury or neuroimaging as a result of cognitive or behavioral deficits from TBI that may limit ability to fully evaluate neurologic status.

Treatment

Medical
- Avoid sedating medications.
  - Histamine-1 blocking agents are sedating.
  - Avoid metoclopramide, which can cause cognitive dysfunction (and extrapyramidal side effects).
  - Tricyclic antidepressants are effectively used for neuropathic pain associated with SCI but can cause sedation and anticholinergic side effects.
  - Use caution with tizanidine for spasticity, which can cause hypotension in an already hypotensive SCI patient.
- Central dysautonomia can be treated with ß-blockers and bromocriptine

Exercises
- Can treat SCI and TBI concomittantly

Modalities
- Heating and cooling modalities should be used with extreme caution in areas of altered sensation.

Surgical
- Neurosurgery

Consults
- Neuropsychology
- Spinal cord medicine

Complications/side effects
- Elevated risk for skin breakdown with sensory and cognitive deficits

Prognosis
- Poorer outcomes are seen in dual diagnosis (SCI with TBI) when compared to single neurologic injury.

Helpful Hints
- Central dysautonomia may present similarly to autonomic dysreflexia (AD). AD is a sudden rise in blood pressure due to an exaggerated reflex to a stimulus originating below the level of the SCI that is seen in injuries T6 or above.
- AD is marked by a hypertension, headaches, mydriasis, flushing and sweating above the lesion, and piloerection and pallor below the lesion.
- In contrast, central dysautonomia is marked by fever, dystonia, extensor posturing, and tachycardia, in addition to the similar sign of hypertension.

Suggested Reading

Bowman BK, Macchiocchi S. Dual diagnosis: Diagnosis, management, and future trends. *Top Spin Cord Inj Rehabil* 2004;10(2):58–68.

Sexual Dysfunction

Description
- Post-TBI issues include erectile dysfunction, decrease in ejaculatory function, decrease in orgasms, decreased libido.
- Hypersexuality is also seen, often manifest with increased masterbatory activity and public masturbation.

Etiology
- Neuroendocrinologic abnormalities
  - Hypopituitarism
  - Hyperprolactinemia
- Medications
  - Antihypertensives
  - Antipsychotics
    - Can cause ejaculatory dysfunction and priapism
- Antidepressants
  - SSRIs cause decreased desire, ejaculatory dysfunction, and orgasmic dysfunction
  - Trazadone is associated with priapism
  - Anxiolytics
  - Sedatives
  - Hormonal agents
- Physical limitations
- Cognitive deficits
- Behavioral dysfunction, including psychosomatic reasons
- Secondary medical conditions
  - Incontinence
  - Diabetes
- Klüver-Bucy syndrome is a behavioral disorder characterized by a heightened sex drive or a tendency to seek sexual stimulation from unusual or inappropriate objects.
- That occurs when both the right and left medial temporal lobes of the brain malfunction. The amygdala has been a particularly implicated brain region in the pathogenesis of this syndrome. Commonly see docility, hyperorality, altered sexuality, visual agnosia.

Risk Factors
- Hypersexuality associated with medial basal-frontal or diencephalic injury

- Right hemisphere lesions associated with greater levels of arousal
- Preinjury alcohol usage

Clinical Features
- After TBI, frequency of intercourse typically decreases.
- Higher rates of erectile dysfunction
- Higher rates of ejaculatory dysfunction
- Higher rates of orgasmic dysfunction
- Sexual dissatisfaction correlates with low self-esteem and decreased interest.
- Greater psychosocial adjustment issues in general are associated with greater sexual dysfunction.

Diagnosis

Differential diagnosis
- None

History
- Identify sexual difficulties
- Inquire about sexual development, sexual beliefs, sexual behaviors, sexual orientation, and current relationship issues.
- Obtain history of sexual, physical, or psychological abuse.
- Obtain detailed review of systems with a focus on symptoms of depression and/or anxiety.
- Substance abuse history

Exam
- Identify physical restraints that may interfere with sexual positioning.
  - Spasticity
  - Contractures
  - Range of motion
- Genital exam
- Sensory exam
- Bulbocavernosus reflex: assess integrity of S2–S5
- Cremasteric reflex: L1 reflex
- Medication review

Testing
- Fasting blood sugar to evaluate for diabetes

- In males: serum testosterone level, LH, FSH, TSH, growth hormone, cortisol
- In females: serum estrogen, LH, FSH, TSH, growth hormone, cortisol
- Strain gauges to assess nocturnal penile erection.
- Vaginal photoplethysmograph devices can assess female arousal.

Pitfalls

- Individual and/or significant other modesty often limits accuracy of evaluation.

Red Flags

- Kluver-Bucy syndrome

Treatment

Medical

- Erectile dysfunction
  - Reduce alcohol consumption
  - Phosphodiesterase inhibitors including sildenafil and vardenafil
  - Topical alprostadil—prostaglandin E1
  - Dopaminergic agents—apomorphine
  - Intracavernosal injection with phentolamine or prostaglandin E1
  - Vacuum constriction erectile devices
- Testosterone replacement

Exercises

- Pelvic floor muscle exercises

Modalities

- None

Surgical

- None

Consults

- Sexual therapist
- Urologist if patient fails conventional therapies for erectile dysfunction

Complications/side effects

- Priapism with PDE-5 inhibitors
- PDE-5 inhibitors contraindicated in patients who are taking nitrites.

Prognosis

- Persistent dysfunction at 3 months is associated with poor long-term outcomes.

Helpful Hints

- Never prescribe 5-phosphodiesterase inhibitors if patient is taking nitrates.

Suggested Reading

Garden FH, Bontke CF, Hoffman M. Sexual function and marital adjustment after traumatic brain injury. *J Head Trauma Rehabil* 1990;5(2):52–59.

Section II: Conditions

Shaken Baby Syndrome

Description
- Inflicted head injury that involves shaking an infant or forcefully striking the infant's head against a surface

Etiology
- Sudden angular deceleration
- Angular decelerative forces usually not present during accidental trauma.
- Perpetrators in descending order of frequency: fathers, boyfriends, female babysitters, mothers

Risk Factors
- Under 3 years of age
- Prior child abuse
- Young parents
- Unstable family situations
- Low socioeconomic status
- Child disability
- Prematurity of child

Clinical Features
- Hallmark of illness is absent to minimal external facial/head trauma but serious intracranial and intraocular bleeding
- 65% to 95% of patients with shaken baby syndrome have retinal hemorrhages.
- Scalp trauma
- Infants may appear lethargic and irritable and may display seizures, abnormal tone, vomiting, feeding difficulties, respiratory difficulties.
- The presence of subarachnoid hemorrhage (SAH) and/or subdural hematoma (SDH) is the most consistent finding.
- Infants may be shaken to the point of apnea, leading to a secondary hypoxic injury.
- Full fontanelles
- May be associated with new and old fractures

Diagnosis

Differential diagnosis
- Accidental injury
- Coagulopathy (hemophilia, Vitamin K deficiency)
- Osteogenesis imperfecta (blue sclera, hearing impairment, hypermobility of joints, bruising, short stature, osteopenia)
- Glutaric aciduria type 1 (hypotonia, dyskinesia, developmental delay, cortical atrophy, subdural hematomas, retinal hemorrhages)

History
- Accurate history is often difficult to obtain.
- Mechanism of injury described may not be consistent with developmental capacity of child.
- Common symptoms include lethargy, irritability, seizures, impaired consciousness, increased/decreased tone, vomiting, feeding difficulties, apnea.

Exam
- Full neurologic examination, including check of fontanelles
- Ophthalmoscopic exam to look for retinal hemorrhages and/or retinal detachment

Testing
- CT scan
  - May see extensive loss of gray–white differentiation and diffuse hypodensity, which is associated with subdural hematoma
  - May see diffuse hypodensity of cerebrum
- MRI for infants with equivocal CT findings
- Skeletal survey
  - Look for multiple posterior or lateral rib fractures and metaphyseal fractures

Pitfalls
- Nontraumatic causes of retinal hemorrhages include SAH, sepsis, coagulopathy, severe hypertension.

Red Flags

- Inconsistencies among caretakers regarding etiology of deficits

Treatment

Medical

- Supportive care
- Intracranial pressure management
- Notify child protective services and the police.

Exercises

- Standard rehabilitation interventions for symptoms

Modalities

- Standard modality interventions for symptoms

Surgical

- Pediatric neurosurgery

Consults

- Neurosurgical consult for large acute hematoma
- Ophthalmologist

Complications/side effects

- None

Prognosis

- 60% of infants who are comatose initially will either die or be left with severe mental retardation, spastic quadriparesis, or other serious motor impairment.

Helpful Hints

- Extracranial injuries are seen in up to 70% of child abuse victims.
- Retinal hemorrhages can also be seen with accidental trauma.
- Retinal hemorrhages are seen for up to 1 month in vaginally delivered babies.
- Epidural hematomas are rarely due to child abuse and usually represent accidental trauma.

Suggested Reading

Di Maio VJM, Altman RL, Kutscher ML, et al. The "Shaken-Baby Syndrome." *N Engl J Med* 1998;339:1329–1330.

Section II: Conditions

Spasticity/Hypertonicity/Rigidity/Clonus

Description

- Hypertonia is an increase in resting muscle tension (tone).
- Spasticity is velocity-dependent hypertonia.
- Rigidity is velocity-independent hypertonia.
- Clonus is a self-sustaining, low-frequency, rhythmic oscillation of an extremity that represents a sustained hyperactive tonic stretch reflex.

Etiology

- Hyperactive tonic stretch reflex most likely secondary to loss-descending cerebral control over spinal motor mechanisms

Risk Factors

- Severe brain injury

Clinical Features

- Spasticity is manifest by excessive resistance to passive stretch of muscle.
- Tendons have low threshold to tapping.
- Examiner may identify "catch" in muscle with rapid, passive stretching.
- Spasticity often interferes with individual's ability to move an extremity either actively or passively; however, hypertonia may actually improve functioning in transfers and gait.
- Spasticity can be exacerbated by local or systemic irritants, such as fractures, urinary tract infections, fecal impaction, pressure ulcers, in-grown toenails.
- Spasticity can lead to permanent loss in range of motion.

Diagnosis

Differential diagnosis

- Rigidity/parkinsonism
- Contractures
- Dystonia
- Paratonia (involuntary variable resistance during passive movement)
- Muscle splinting due to painful muscle spasm
- Medication side effects (antipsychotics)

History

- Identify prior evidence of increased tone.
- Identify risk factors for spasticity triggers.

Exam

- Check passive and active range of motion (ROM) of extremities.
- Evaluate motor strength.
- Evaluate deep tendon reflexes.
- Assess spasticity with standardized measurement tool, eg,
  - Modified Ashworth Scale—most commonly used scale
    - 0 = no increase in tone
    - 1 = slightly increased tone with a catch/release or minimal resistance at terminal ROM
    - 1+ = slightly increased tone with a catch, followed by minimal resistance through the remainder (less than half) of the ROM
    - 2+ = increased tone through most of the ROM, but affected part easily moved
    - 3 = considerably increased tone; passive motion difficult
    - 4 = affected part rigid

Pitfalls

- Joint contractures or extremity internal derangements/fractures can mimic or exacerbate spasticity.
- Muscle or joint pain can mimic or exacerbate spasticity.

Red Flags

- Worsening spasticity can signal a new or worsening brain lesion, including hydrocephalus.
- Worsening spasticity can signal infection, wound, or other trigger.

Treatment

- Indications for treatment include functional deficits (including hygiene), pain, poor positioning, pain, and insomnia.

Medical

- Systemic medications—see following section
- Focal medications
  - Phenol injection
    - Used for mixed nerve blockade or motor point block
    - Can cause dysesthesias and sensory loss when used as a neurolytics agent

– Botulinum toxin
  ○ Off-label use to treat focal spasticity

Exercises/rehabilitation
- Stretching and positioning
- Serial casting and splinting

Modalities
- Cryotherapy
- Hot packs
- Functional electrical stimulation

Surgical
- Intrathecal baclofen
- Tendon transfers, muscle lengthening, rhizotomy, myelotomy

Consults
- Neurosurgery
- Orthopedic surgery

Complications/side effects
- Excessive treatment may result in weakness/hypotonia with a decrease in function
- Medication specific side effects

Prognosis
- No specific association between spasticity and outcome
- While reports of spasticity aiding in functional mobility persist, limited evidence to support a positive association between spasticity and outcome
- Spasticity promotes maintenance of muscle bulk/mass

Helpful Hints
- IV physostigmine 1 to 2 mg can be used in baclofen overdose.
- Combination therapy with two oral agents often indicated in severe spasticity.
- Early use (within first month) of focal injectables should be considered with severe spasticity.

Suggested Reading
Gracies JM, Elovic E, McGuire JR, Nance P, Simpson DM. Traditional pharmacologic treatments for spasticity. Part II: Systemic treatments. In: Mayer NH, Simpson DM, eds. *Spasticity Etiology, Evaluation, Management and the Role of Botulinim Toxin.* New York: WE MOVE; 2002.

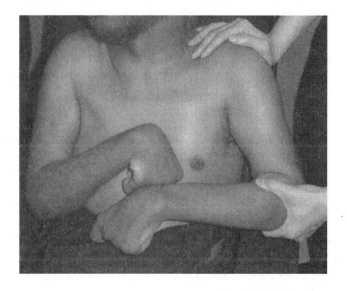

A familiar upper motor neuron pattern of upper limb deformity: adducted/internally rotated shoulder; flexed elbow; pronated forearm; bent wrist; clenched fist; thumb-in-palm. (With permission from Zasler ND, Katz DI, Zafonte RD. *Brain Injury Medicine: Principles and Practice.* New York: Demos Medical Publishing; 2007.)

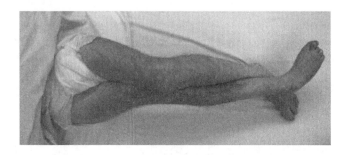

A familiar UMN pattern of lower limb deformity: flexed hip, adducted (scissoring thighs); flexed knee; stiff knee; equinovarus foot. (With permission from Zasler ND, Katz DI, Zafonte RD. *Brain Injury Medicine: Principles and Practice.* New York: Demos Medical Publishing; 2007.)

Section II: Conditions

Tinnitus

Description
- Perception of ringing, high-pitched whining, or buzzing within the ear without a corresponding external sound
- Can be intermittent or continuous
- Can cause great distress to patient
- Can be objective (audible to anyone, including affected individual) or subjective (audible only to affected individual)
- Objective tinnitus is extremely rare.

Etiology
- Loss or malfunctioning of inner ear hair cells
- Objective muscular tinnitus: stapedius or tensor tympani myoclonus
- Objective vascular tinnitus: aberrance of carotid artery that causes turbulence as it passes near the ear or due to venous hum

Risk Factors
- Ear infections
- Sensorineural hearing loss
- Exposure to loud noises

Clinical Features
- Ringing, buzzing, whining, or whooshing sound heard within the ear without corresponding external sound
- May be pulsatile in nature due to altered blood flow through the ear
- Often exacerbated in stressful situations
- May be cyclical with female menstrual periods

Diagnosis

Differential diagnosis
- Side effect of excessive aspirin use
- Side effect of quinidine
- Acoustic neuromas
- Meniere disease
- Mercury or lead poisoning
- Multiple sclerosis

History
- Question about concomitant hearing loss
- Medication history
- Depression symptoms
- Tinnitus Handicap Inventory: can quantify tinnitus and how it affects daily living

Exam
- Auscultate neck for bruits
- Auscultation of jugular vein for venous hum
- Otoscopic exam to assess for excessive ear wax and integrity of tympanic membrane
- Special stethoscopes needed to detect objective tinnitus

Testing
- Audiology screen to assess for concomitant hearing loss
- CT scan of ossicles
- MRI/MRA for pulsatile tinnitus
- MRI for unilateral tinnitus to assess for acoustic neuroma

Pitfalls
- Multiple causes for tinnitus make identifying etiologies extremely difficult.

Red Flags
- Pulsatile tinnitus may be a symptom of carotid artery aneurysm or dissection.
- Unilateral tinnitus
- Tinnitus with vertigo

Treatment

Medical
- Avoid ototoxic medications (aminoglycosides, chloramphenicol, erythromycin, tetracycline, vancomycin, methotrexate, cisplatin, vincristine, bumetanide, furosemide, quinine).
- Biofeedback
- Treatment of depression

- Correct hearing loss with hearing aids
- Homeopathic therapy, including ginkgo biloba and niacin, has been used, but without supporting evidence.

Exercises
- None

Modalities
- Electrical stimulation of inner ear (controversial)
- Tinnitus maskers
- White noise at night can help sleep.
- Acupuncture may have positive effect initially.

Surgical
- Cochlear implant

Consults
- Otolaryngology
- Audiology

Prognosis
- More than 95% of tinnitus after TBI resolves in the first 4 weeks after injury.
- If present > 3 months, it is unlikely to completely resolve, even with treatment.

Helpful Hints
- There is limited evidence to support treatments for tinnitus.

Suggested Reading
Marion MS, Cevette MJ. Tinnitus. *Mayo Clin Proced* 1991;66:614–620.

Tremors

Description
- Tremor is an unintentional, somewhat rhythmic, muscle movement involving to-and-fro movements (oscillations) of one or more parts of the body.
- Most common movement disorders in TBI is an intention tremor. Parkinsonian, cerebellar, and dystonic tremors can also occur.
- Seen in approximately 8% of patients with severe TBI and 1.3% with moderate-mild TBI.
- Intention tremors are tremors that are worse during intention, (eg, as the patient's finger approaches a target), including cerebellar disorders.

Etiology
- Pathophysiology of tremors after TBI is not fully elucidated and may have more to do with connection pathways (eg, associated with diffuse axonal injury [DAI], lesions in dentatothalamic tract are associated with delayed tremor).
- Majority of patients have a history of deceleration trauma.

Risk Factors
- Presence of generalized edema on CT scan is significantly associated with occurrence of a movement disorder.
- Presence of DAI on CT/MRI.

Clinical Features
- May be apparent soon after injury, but can occur years later
- High amplitude postural and kinetic tremors are the most disabling, as they interfere with mobility.
- May be interrupted by myoclonic type movements
- May also be present at rest, resembling a parkinsonian tremor
- Predominately affects the upper extremity
- Rarely an isolated symptom; often associated with psychological dysfunction, cognitive dysfunction, hemiparesis, dysarthria, oculomotor dysfunction, and/or truncal ataxia.

Diagnosis

Differential diagnosis
- Myoclonus
- Asterixis
- Clonus
- Epilepsia partialis continua
- Hyperthyroidism
- Ballism
- Chorea
- Delirium tremens (acute)

History
- Tremor duration, severity, exacerbating/relieving factors
- History of tremor
- Family history of tremor
- History of seizure disorder
- Alcohol/illicit drug usage

Exam
- Examine during sleep, rest, and when moving.

Testing
- Thyroid function panel
- Liver function panel

Pitfalls
- Cerebellar dysfunction may be labeled as tremors.

Red Flags
- Seizure disorder must be ruled out.

Treatment

Medical
- Parkinsonian tremor drug treatment involves levodopa and/or dopamine-like drugs such as pergolide mesylate, bromocriptine mesylate, and ropinirole.
- Other drugs used to lessen parkinsonian tremor include amantadine hydrochloride and anticholinergic drugs.
- Essential tremor may be treated with propranolol, nadolol, or other β- blockers, and primidone.
- Cerebellar tremor typically does not respond to medical treatment.
- Dystonic tremor may respond to Valium, anticholinergic drugs, and intramuscular injections of botulinum toxin. Botulinum toxin is also prescribed to treat voice and head tremors and several movement disorders.

Exercises/rehabilitation
- Weighted utensils
- Weights on wrists or fingers

Modalities
- None

Surgical
- Ablative functional stereotactic surgery of the ventrolateral thalamus and subthalamic region is used for recalcitrant tremor. Tremor at rest usually completely abolished. Reduction in postural and kinetic tremor. May show increase in dystonic posture, worsening of dysarthria
- Thalamic deep brain stimulation (DBS) is less effective for posttraumatic tremor vs parkinsonian or essential tremor.

Consults
- Neurology for nonresponders to first-line agents.
- Neurosurgery for severe tremor interfering with function and not responding to medication

Complications/side effects
- Medication effects
- Risks of surgery/DBS

Prognosis
- Tremors associated with mild-moderate TBI usually do not require therapy and usually subside spontaneously.
- No clear association between tremor and short- or long-term outcomes.

Helpful Hints
- Essential tremor may be accompanied by mild gait disturbance.
- The efficacy of botulinum toxin is limited due to the high number of muscles that must be treated for satisfactory outcome.

Suggested Reading
Obeso JA, Narbona J. Posttraumatic tremor and myoclonic jerking. *J Neurol Neurosurg Psychiatr* 1993;46:788.

Clinical presentation of patients with posttraumatic dystonia. (A) Patient with right-sided hemidystonia and cervical dystonia, before thalamotomy. (B) Same patient at long-term follow-up after left-sided thalamotomy. (C) Dystonic posture of right hand. (D) Left-sided dystonia with superimposed athetotic movements. (E) Right-sided hemidystonia. (F) Typical increase of dystonia upon intended movement. (With permission from Krauss JK, Mohadjer M, Braus DF, Wakhloo AK, Nobbe F, Mundinger F. Dystonia following head trauma—a report of nine patients and review of the literature. *Mov Disord* 1992;7:263–272.)

Vegetative State, Persistent

Description
- No awareness of self or environment with inability to interact with others or the environment
- The capacity for spontaneous or stimulus produced arousal is preserved.
- Labeled "persistent" when no improvement after 12 months

Etiology
- Brainstem injury
- Diffuse axonal injury
- Anoxic brain injury

Risk Factors
- Coma
- Progressive degenerative disorder
- Progressive metabolic disorder
- Paramedial thalamic damage
- Laminar cortical necrosis

Clinical Features
- No purposeful behaviors; however, reflex behaviors (eg, chewing, smiling) are preserved.
- May see sleep–wake cycles

Diagnosis

Differential diagnosis
- Coma
- Minimally conscious state
- Locked-in syndrome
- Subclinical seizures
- Catatonia
- Akinetic mutism

History
- Investigate other causes of decreased arousal, including medication and seizures.

Exam
- No purposeful behaviors noted to visual, auditory, tactile, or painful stimuli.
- Assess integrity of brainstem.
  - Pupillary response
  - Ocular movements
  - Oculovestibular reflexes
  - Corneal response
- Assess for pathologic posturing.
- Assess cortical functioning.
  - Tracking
  - Simple verbal commands
  - Noxious stimulation localization
- Optimize patient-related factors for arousal.
- Minimalize environmental distractions and provide adequate lighting.
- Use simple language.
- Choose simple commands that patient will be able to perform within their motor capacity.
- Avoid asking patient to squeeze hand or blink eyes, as these can be reflexic actions.
  - Purposeful movements include tracking or reaching for object in visual field.
- Look for purposeful behavior.
  - Try placing object in patient's hand, and see if they manipulate it.
  - Smiling or crying at picture of family member
  - Bringing toothbrush to mouth
  - Bringing hairbrush to hair
- Assess integrity of CNS
  - Brainstem evaluation includes pupillary reflexes, ocular movements, oculovestibular reflexes, gag reflex.
- May need serial assessment, as patient may be inconsistent
- Standardized rating scales: JFK Coma Recovery Scale, Coma-Near Coma Scale

Testing
- EEG if seizure activity suspected
- Evoked potentials (VER, BAER, SSEPP, MEP) to assess ability to perceive stimuli
- Functional neuroimaging (fMRI, fPET) to assess for cognitive functioning
- The Coma-Near Coma Scale is a good monitoring tool that can be performed by a variety of clinicians.

Pitfalls
- Encephalomalacia on brain imaging is common after severe TBI with vegetative state and may be misinterpreted as hydrocephalus.

Red Flags
- Subtle declines in arousal level may indicate medical complication (eg, UTI); however, they may be hard to

determine without uniform measurement system in place.

Treatment

Medical
- Sensory stimulation to improve arousal level
- Maintain range of motion
- Management of common comorbidities (spasticity, heterotopic ossification, pressure ulcer, joint flexibility)
- Amantadine is first-line agent, but limited research support
- Bromocriptine: case reports demonstrate recovery of speech.

Exercises
- None

Modalities
- Median nerve (noxious) stimulation advocated but limited scientific support

Surgical
- Deep brain stimulation, but limited scientific support

Consults
- Neurology if suspect seizure activity limiting arousal
- Neurosurgery if suspect hydrocephalus limiting arousal

Complications/side effects
- Amantadine lowers the seizure threshold and should be used with care.

Prognosis
- Better prognosis for those with traumatic vs nontraumatic injury

- If unconscious at 1 month, 33% will regain consciousness by 3 months postinjury, 46% by 6 months, and 53% by 1 year.
- If unconscious at 3 months, only 35% chance of recovery by 1 year.
- If unconscious at 6 months postinjury, only 16% chance of consciousness at 1 year.
- Prognosis for consciousness very poor if consciousness not present by 1 year postinjury.
- 50% of patients will be severely disabled and 33% moderately disabled by 12 months postinjury.
- If > 40 years old, worse functional outcome
- Mortality rates are higher for patients that have been in a VS for at least 1 month
  - 82% mortality at 3 years
  - 95% mortality at 5 years

Helpful Hints
- The term vegetative state does not imply irreversibility.
- There may be significant variability in the level of arousal throughout the day related to fluctuating cognitive function or sleep–wake cycling.
- Consistent monitoring of cognitive/arousal status using standardized scales (CNC, JFK Coma Recovery Scale) is recommended to uniformly assess status.
- Significant (consistent) worsening on standardized scales may indicate evidence of medical decline (eg, urinary tract infection) rather than an acute cerebral process.

Suggested Reading
Multi-Society Task Force Report on PVS. Medical aspects of the persistent vegetative state. *NEJM* 1994;330:1499–1508, 1572–1579.

Section II: Conditions

Vision Deficits

Description
- Visual deficits after TBI are common and may range from difficulties with the functioning of the eye (asthenopia) to central interpretation of vision (perception).

Etiology
- Retinal damage
- Cranial nerve injury (see chapters discussing Cranial Nerve Deficits, pages 60–69)
- Midbrain damage
  - Approximately 20% of fibers conveying retinal information arrive at the midbrain and interact with proprioceptive and vestibular fibers.
- Occipital lobe damage
- Visual field deficits are due to insults to the visual pathways
  - Optic nerve: complete unilateral blindness
  - Optic chiasma: bitemporal hemianopsia
  - Optic tract: complete ipsilateral homonymous hemianopsia
  - Superior lateral geniculate tract and/or inferior lateral geniculate tract: ipsilateral inferior homonymous hemianopsia

Risk Factors
- TBI with penetrating fragments or facial fractures may be associated with globe injuries.
- Blunt trauma to occiput most commonly associated with occipital lobe visual deficits

Clinical Features
- Most common visual complaint is blurred vision, followed by diplopia.
- Most common visual field deficit is compression of peripheral fields, followed by homonymous hemianopsia.
- Other complaints include difficulty shifting gaze, photophobia, difficulty tracking, and visual midline shift syndrome.
- The altered perception of the visual midline seen with homonymous hemianopsia may result in a shifting of the patient's midline orientation that will result in difficulty in functioning.

Diagnosis

Differential diagnosis
- Focal globe(s) injury
  - Detached retina
  - Dislocated or fractured optic lens
- Retained contact lens
- Cortical blindness

History
- Premorbid visual difficulties
- Premorbid use of glasses, contacts
- History of myopia corrective surgery

Exam
- Cranial nerve examination
- Extraocular movements
- Visual acuity
- Convergence
- Accommodation
- Visual fields
- Fundoscopic examination

Testing
- Visual evoked potentials
- Precise visual field assessment via computerized threshold perimetry

Pitfalls
- CT and MRI often cannot detect lesions specific to the oculomotor cranial nerves.

Red Flags
- Eye pain may indicate elevated intraocular pressures.
- Acutely declining vision

Treatment

Medical
- Glaucoma treatment as indicated

Exercises/rehabilitation
- Visual (neuro-optometric) rehabilitation

Modalities
- Orthoptic, such as Fresnel prism lenses
- Patching or use of translucent lenses or spot patches for diplopia

Surgical
- None

Consults
- Neuro-ophthalmology

Complications/side effects
- None

Prognosis
- If symptoms are not improving by 12 months post-TBI, unlikely to fully recover

Helpful Hints
- Patients tend to lean away from side of visual loss in homonymous hemianopsia.
- Monocular diplopia is a rare disorder caused by focal damage to one eye/globe.
- Terson syndrome is the occurrence of vitreous hemorrhage in association with subarachnoid hemorrhage.
- Anton syndrome (cortical blindness)—clinical evidence of blindness or near blindness; however, patient is unaware of limitations

Suggested Reading
Padula WV, Shapiro JB. Head injury causing post-trauma vision syndrome. *New Eng J Optometry* 1988; December:16–2.

Visual Perceptual Deficits

Description
- Visual-perceptual disorders include unilateral spatial inattention (neglect), cortical blindness, impaired color perception, visual agnosia, visual-spatial disorders, and visual-constructive disorders.
- Cortical, or central, blindness (Anton syndrome) is a primary sensory disorder with complete or near complete loss of vision without awareness of the impaired individual.
- Color imperception is defective color awareness after a brain injury.
- Color agnosia describes the inability to name colors correctly and is often accompanied by the syndrome of alexia without agraphia.
- Visual agnosia is the failure to recognize familiar objects and their function (faces, letters) despite intact visual spatial processing and intellectual function.
- Facial agnosia (prosopagnosia) is usually seen in combination with other deficits including visual-spatial disorientation, color imperception, and left upper quadrant visual field loss.

Etiology
- Cortical blindness is due to bilateral cerebral destruction of the visual projection cortex (area 17).
- Color imperception is associated with right hemisphere or bilateral occipital lobe lesions.
- Color agnosia is more common with left hemispheric lesions.
- Visual agnosia is associated with bilateral lesions to the visual associative areas (areas 18 and 19).

Risk Factors
- N/A

Clinical Features
- Cortical blindness: individual may report blurry vision or may be unaware of impairment.
- Color imperception: individual may report colors appear "muddy."
- Visual agnosia: lack of recognition of common objects including faces (facial agnosia), perceiving only one element of an object and not the whole object
- In visual agnosia, an individual can typically recognize the object by touch or by hearing how it used.

Diagnosis

Differential diagnosis
- Dementia

History
- Premorbid visual deficits

Exam
- Visual acuity
- Visual field deficits
- Color discrimination tests

Testing
- No standardized tests for agnosia
- Place common objects in front of subject. Subject must name the object and describe its function.
- Facial agnosia can be tested by presenting individual with photographs of famous world figures, actors, or family members.

Pitfalls
- Language deficits, particularly word finding difficulty, that would impede naming objects

Red Flags
- Worsening visual perception may indicate either an acute intracranial abnormality or a systemic cause of worsening cognition

Treatment

Medical
- None

Exercises
- For partial cortical blindness, a headlamp can be used to improve visual localization.

- With color imperception, treatment tasks should initially involve materials with sharp color contrasts and then progress to materials with less contrast.
- For visual agnosia, tactile input with simultaneous visual input can be encouraged as a compensation technique.

Modalities
- None

Surgical
- None

Consults
- Vision rehabilitation specialist

Complications/side effects
- None

Prognosis
- Initial deficits are associated with worse functional outcomes and longer acute hospital stays.
- Persistent deficits at 3 months are indicative of poor long-term recovery and of overall poor prognosis.

Helpful Hints
- Total loss of color perception is rare.
- Visual agnosia can only be diagnosed if visual acuity is intact and language skills are intact (no word finding difficulty).

Suggested Reading
Hellerstein LF, Fishman B. Vision therapy and occupational therapy: An integrated approach. *J Behav Optom* 1990;42:312–322.

Section II: Conditions

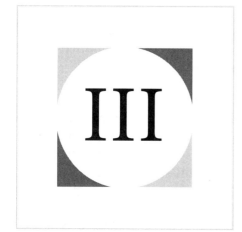

Interventions

Acute Management of Mild Traumatic Brain Injury

Description
- Focus is on patient education (common symptoms and excellent prognosis) and symptom management.

Key Principles
- Airway, breathing, and circulation should be attended to prior to other injuries.
- Computerized tomography (CT) scan of head is cornerstone of evaluation when at least one of the following is present: loss of consciousness, posttraumatic amnesia (PTA), confusion, impaired alertness.
- Neuropsychological testing may assist in diagnostic workup.
- Identify secondary causes of injury including hypotension and hypoxia.
- Blood alcohol levels should be tested in all patients.

Indications
- Comprehensive evaluation and close monitoring are appropriate.

Contraindications
- Rapid return to activity (except contact sports) is appropriate.

Special Considerations
- Patients with any of the following symptoms should have more detailed testing (CT scan):
  - Focal neurologic deficit
  - Asymmetric pupils
  - Multiple trauma (especially if painful injuries are distracting)
  - Loss of consciousness
  - Vomiting
  - Posttraumatic seizure
  - Skull fractures
  - Age > 60 or < 2 years
  - Suspected child abuse
  - PTA
  - Progressively worsening headache
  - History of bleeding disorder or taking anticoagulation

Key Procedural Steps
- Acute trauma assessment and management
- Assessment of presence and duration of loss of consciousness, PTA, and retrograde amnesia
- Assessment of posttraumatic symptoms
- Pain assessment
- Mental status exam
- Full neurologic exam including Glasgow Coma Scale
- Blood alcohol level
- Urine toxicology screen
- Neuroimaging if indicated
- Analgesics for pain

Anticipated Problems
- Analgesics may interfere with mental status exam.
- Symptoms (headache, dizziness, insomnia, cognitive deficits, behavioral disturbances) are common in the first 24 hours to 2 weeks but are typically self-limited in the first month with common interventions (medication, counseling, education). Persistent problems at 4 weeks should be aggressively managed.

Helpful Hints
- All patients with loss of consciousness or posttraumatic sensorium disturbance should undergo CT scanning of the head.

Acute Management of Moderate to Severe Traumatic Brain Injury

Description
- Refers to interval between head injury and eventual discharge from acute care

Key Principles
- Focuses on prevention of secondary brain injury

Indications
- All individuals who sustain a moderate or severe TBI should be acutely managed in a level I trauma center.
- Inpatient, interdisciplinary rehabilitation care is appropriate for all individuals with disability after TBI that cannot be safely managed at home and who are able to participate in treatments (Rancho Los Amigos level III or higher).

Contraindications
- None

Special Considerations
- Intoxicated individuals need special attention even without signs of external injury.
- Key procedural steps
- Airway, breathing, and circulation should be assessed first in a patient with suspected brain injury.
- Full cervical spine immobilization should be performed.
- Patient should be transported to a center where TBI is managed in entirety.
- Glasgow Coma Scale should be used to assess the patient.
- Any loss of consciousness should be recorded.
- Posttraumatic amnesia should be assessed and recorded.
- Anticoagulant use should be assessed if possible.
- Avoid strong analgesia for headache until assessment in the emergency room.
- Blood alcohol levels should be tested.

- Labs should include complete metabolic panel, complete blood count, type and screen for blood products, coagulation profile, and arterial blood gas.
- Full neurologic exam
- Correct hypovolemia, hypotension, and hypoxia.
- Acute short-term hyperventilation is a short-term life-saving intervention for individuals demonstrating signs of uncal herniation.
- With deepening coma or pupillary inequality, use of osmotic agents like mannitol should be considered to help lower the intracranial pressure (ICP).
- Posttraumatic seizure prophylaxis should be initiated as soon as possible.
- Imaging should be done as early as possible.
- Nutrition should be initiated within 2–3 days of injury.

Anticipated Problems
- Raised ICP
- Patients with severe TBI require airway management.

Helpful Hints
- Avoid any nasogastric tubes if basilar skull fracture suspected. Tube can penetrate cranium.
- The classic "lucid interval" associated with epidural hematoma only occurs 30% of the time.
- Epidural hematomas > 30 cm in volume usually need to be evacuated surgically.
- Nutritional needs are estimated to increased > 40% in the severely injured TBI patient.

Suggested Reading
Iverson GL. Outcome from mild traumatic brain injury. *Arch Clin Neuropsychol* 2000;15:643–648.

Agitation: Medications to Treat

Drug	Mechanism of Action	Dosing	Advantages	Disadvantages
Haloperidol	Dopamine antagonist	2 mg initially 10–20 mg daily max dose	Can be given IM or IV Rapid onset of action ~30 minutes	May prolong brain recovery May cause extrapyramidal symptoms May lead to akathisia (motor restlessness) Prolong QT interval May lower seizure threshold Neuroleptic malignant syndrome
Lorezapam	GABA agonist	1–2 mg doses	Only benzodiazepine with rapid IM absorption Few drug–drug interactions	Can exacerbate confusion and cause further agitation May be detrimental to brain injury recovery
Olanzepine	Dopamine and serotonin antagonist	Start 5 mg orally Max oral 10 mg. 10 mg IM for severe agitation. May repeat ×2 every 3 hours	Oral and IM preparations Rapid onset of action	Do not coadminister with benzodiazepines
Propanolol	β-Blocker	Start 60 mg Max 420 mg	Helps treat symptoms of hyperadrenalism	Side effects include sedation, hypotension, and bradycardia
Methylphenidate	Facilitates dopamine and norepinephrine transmission	Start 5 mg twice daily Average dose 20–30 mg daily Max 60 mg daily	Helps with concentration	Cautions in patients with cardiovascular dysfunction
Amantadine	Facilitates dopamine transmission	Start 50 mg twice daily Max 400 mg	May enhance recovery	May lead to anxiety or visual hallucinations
Valproic Acid	Anticonvulsant	Start 10 mg/kg/day Max 60 mg/kg/day	Usually effective within 1 week No significant effect on neuropsychological testing	Can cause nausea if not dosed at mealtimes May lead to pancreatitis or hepatitis
Carbamezapine	Anticonvulsant	Start 200 mg twice daily Max 1200 mg daily	Particularly good effect for irritability and disinhibition	May cause motor slowing Can cause aplastic anemia, hyponatremia, and renal failure Must monitor serum levels Look out for Stephens-Johnson syndrome

Drug	Mechanism of Action	Dosing	Advantages	Disadvantages
Buspirone	Serotonin agonist	Start 7.5 mg twice daily Max 60 mg daily	Does not interact with other drugs Nonsedating Significant anxiolytic properties	May induce seizures
Sertraline	SSRI	Start 50 mg daily Max 200 mg daily	Helps treat emotional lability	2 weeks for clinical effectiveness
Citalopram	SSRI	Start 20 mg daily Max 60 mg daily	Helps treat emotional lability	2 weeks for clinical effectiveness
Trazadone	Serotonin agonist	Start 50–100 mg.	Causes sedation and can promote sleep at night	May cause serotonin syndrome in patients on SSRIs Anticholinergic symptoms Priapism

IM = intramuscularly, IV = intravenously, SSRI = selective serotonin reuptake inhibitor.

Suggested Reading

Lombard LA, Zafonte RD. Agitation after traumatic brain injury: Considerations and treatment options. *Am J Phys Med Rehabil* 2005;84:797–812.

Section III: Interventions

Complementary Alternative Medicine

Description
- The use of nontraditional medicine to treat the sequela of traumatic brain injury

Key Principles
- Medications used to enhance cognition include choline, phosphatidylcholine, CDP-choline, gingko biloba, pyritonol, piracetam
- Kava contains centrally acting muscle relaxants and anticonvulsants and has been used to alleviate anxiety and insomnia.
- Picamilon is a niacin analogue that reportedly reduces anxiety and hyperesthesia.
- Valerian reportedly improves sleep quality and decreases sleep latency.
- St. John's wort (hypericum) has been used to treat mild to moderate depression.
- Gingko biloba may improve dizziness, nystagmus, and smooth pursuit gain.
- Pyritinol may improve vertigo.
- Piracetam may improve vertigo of central origin.

Indications
- Cognitive deficits
- Depression
- Sleep disturbance

Contraindications
- Drug interactions with tradition medications are not uncommon.

- Many complementary alternative medications are not standardized or regulated.

Special Considerations
- Gingko biloba may be associated with increased bleeding risk, as it has been shown to inhibit platelet activation factor.
- A Valerian withdrawal syndrome has been described as that involved delirium.
- Valerian has a very unpleasant odor that may be disliked by patients.

Key Procedural Steps
- N/A

Anticipated Problems
- Side effects associated with gingko biloba include nausea, headache, diarrhea, allergy, restlessness, and sleep disturbance.

Helpful Hints
- CAM represents a potential area of clinical intervention for TBI, but research is lacking and safety concerns must be high.

Suggested Reading
McElligott J, Davis AM, Hecht JS, Kothari S, Muenz JA, Wang GG. Complementary and alternative medicine. In: Zasler ND, Katz DI, Zafonte RD, eds. *Brain Injury Medicine*. New York: Demos; 2007:1061–1082.

Computer-Based Cognitive Therapy

Description
- Computer-based programs that emphasize memory, thinking, and information processes—designed to facilitate cognitive recovery after brain injury
- Use of computers in cognitive therapy is an established rehabilitation process.
- Driving inventories are available that help identify individuals who are not safe to drive before an on-road test.
- Simulated driving computerized programs are available to aid in driving retraining.

Key Principles
- Use of computerized attentional training
- Computer games typically require attention, concentration, visual scanning, and simultaneous processing, all skills that are typically affected after brain injury.
- Limited research evidence to support usage.

Indications
- Deficits in attention
- Memory impairments
- Computerized cognitive prosthetic (ie, visually mediated communication system for those individuals with a nonfluent aphasia, recording or storage systems, dictation or speech synthesis systems, electronic planning systems)

- Driving retraining
- Math retraining

Contraindications
- Limited evidence to support usage
- Limited hand dexterity limits use of standard keyboard (consider visually controlled system)
- Vegetative state
- Minimally conscious state

Special Considerations
- May have a role as adjuvant therapy but inferior to therapist-directed care

Key Procedural Steps
- Close monitoring of use and efficacy

Anticipated Problems
- Individualized treatments are challenging.

Suggested Reading
Chen SHA, Thomas JD, Glueckauf RL, Bracy OL. The effectiveness of computer-assisted cognitive rehabilitation for persons with traumatic brain injury. *Brain Inj* 1997;11(3):197–209.

Constraint-Induced Movement Therapy

Description
- Constraint-induced movement therapy (CIMT) is a rehabilitation method that focuses on motor recovery of a hemiparetic limb(s) through forced use while the more functional limb is restrained.
- CIMT is based on the principle of "learned nonuse" of a weak upper limb.
- Forced-use therapy entails similar principles to CIMT, but rather than constraining the intact limb, it is used to assist in functional activities, specifically ambulation. It may also be performed when neither limb is intact (as in paraplegia).
- Forced-use therapy may be performed on a treadmill with therapists assisting the weakened limb and an overhead support system to maintain the patient upright.
- Forced-use therapy may be performed using a robotic-assisted treadmill platform (eg, the Lokomat).
- Therapeutic effect is thought to be due to cortical reorganization related to repeated stimulation of peripheral sensory and motor fibers.

Key Principles
- Unaffected arm is restrained with a mitt, sling, or glove for 90% of waking hours for a 2–3 week period.
- In the classic model, an individual will participate in 6–7 hours of therapy daily in addition to performing activities of daily living in the home setting.
- Treadmill-assisted or Lokomat therapy is performed at least 1 hour/day, 5 days/week for 12–24 weeks.

Indications
- Individuals with hemiparesis but some retained ability to extend wrist (20° wrist extension) and fingers (able to release grip from a tennis ball placed in the hand)
- Individuals with lower extremity weakness who can tolerate upright positioning and repeated lower extremity motion (ie, minimal contractures, minimal increased tone)

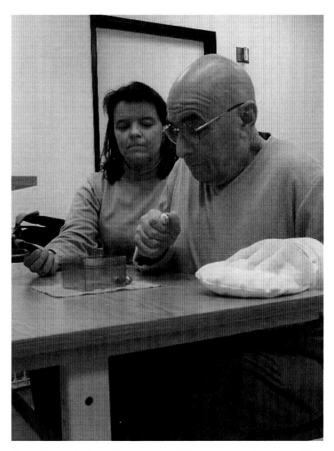

Constraint-induced movement therapy is a therapeutic intervention where use of a constraint device and intensive task practice is used to promote upper limb recovery in individuals with hemiparesis. (With permission from Zasler ND, Katz DI, Zafonte RD. *Brain Injury Medicine: Principles and Practice.* New York: Demos Medical Publishing; 2007.)

Contraindications
- Inadequate balance while wearing restraint
- No hand or wrist active movement
- Completely flaccid hemiparetic limb
- Moderate to severe cognitive impairment
- Severe spasticity, limiting joint movement

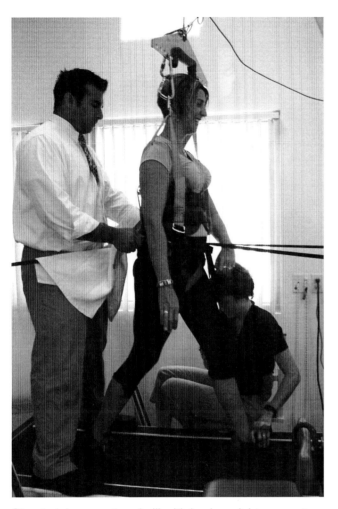

Step training on a treadmill with body weight support is an example of intense, task-specific training that incorporates the repetitive practice of walking. (With permission from Zasler ND, Katz DI, Zafonte RD. *Brain Injury Medicine: Principles and Practice* New York: Demos Medical Publishing; 2007.)

Special Considerations

- Requires a significant amount of therapy time
- Not typically used during the acute rehabilitation setting, as this time is focused on gross mobility, not fine motor skills as much.
- Many individuals have difficulty completing the therapeutic schedule due to time and physical demands.
- Limited long-term carryover

Key Procedural Steps

- Requires regimented approach, dedicated patient, and significant resources
- Limited third-party reimbursement available

Anticipated Problems

- May see improvements on rehabilitation outcome measures that do translate into real-life situations

Helpful Hints

- Motivated patients will see benefits; however, applying improvements to daily activities is key to long-term durability of results.

Suggested Reading

Wolf SL, Lecraw DE, Barton LA, Jann BBL. Forced use of hemiplegic upper extremities to reverse the effect of learned nonuse among chronic stroke and head-injured patients. *Exp Neurol* 1989;104:125–132.

Depression: Medications to Treat

Drug	Dosing	Mechanism of Action	Advantages	Disadvantages
Fluoxetine (Prozac)	20–80 mg/day	SSRI	Low anticholinergic side effects	Many drug–drug interactions Sexual side effects
Sertraline (Zoloft)	50–200 mg/day	SSRI	Low anticholinergic side effects	Of the SSRIs, least likely to have a cytochrome-related drug interaction. Sexual side effects
Paroxetine (Paxil)	20–50 mg/day	SSRI	Helps with anxiety	Needs to be discontinued slowly Sexual side effects
Citalopram (Celexa)	20–60 mg/day	SSRI	Few drug interactions	Sexual side effects
Escitalopram (Lexapro)	10–20 mg/day	SSRI	Quicker onset of action (1–2 weeks)	Sexual side effects
Fluvoxamine (Luvox)	50–250 mg/day	SSRI	Helpful for anxiety and OCD	Potentiates theophyllines Sexual side effects
Buproprion (Wellbutrin)	225–450 mg/day in 3 doses	Inhibits reuptake of serotonin and NE	Less sexual side effects	Lowers seizure threshold Contraindicated in eating disorders
Mirtazapine (Remeron)	15–45 mg at bedtime	Potentiates NE and serotonin	Less sexual side effects Can promote sleep	Very sedating Weight gain Risk of agranulocytosis
Venlaxafine (Effexor XR)	75–225 mg daily if XR	Serotonin and NE reuptake inhibitor	Few drug interactions Helps with pain	Lowers seizure threshold Increases level of Haldol
Duloxetine (Cymbalta)	40–60 mg/day in 1–2 doses	Inhibits reuptake of serotonin and NE	Helps with neuropathic pain and fibromyalgia	Contraindicated in uncontrolled narrow angle glaucoma Caution with hepatic impairment
Amitriptyline	25–300 mg/day	Tricyclic antidepressant	Helps with neuropathic pain Improved sleep	Orthostatic hypotension Arrhythmias Can be lethal in overdose
Nortriptyline	25–150 mg/day	Tricyclic antidepressant	Helps with neuropathic pain Improved sleep	Orthostatic hypotension Arrhythmias Can be lethal in overdose

NE = norepinephrine, OCD = obsessive-compulsive disorder, SSRI = selective serotonin reuptake inhibitor, XR = extended release

Suggested Reading

Fann JR, Uomoto JM, Katon WJ. Sertraline in the treatment of major depression following mild traumatic brain injury. *J Neuropschiatr Clin Neurosci* 2000;12:226–232.

Disability Determination

Description
- American Medical Association definition of disability: "an alteration of an individual's capacity to meet personal, social, or occupational demands or statutory or regulatory requirements because of an impairment"
- Social Security Administration definition of disability: "inability to engage in any substantial gainful activity...by reason of any medically determinable physical or mental impairment that can be expected to result in death or that has lasted or can be expected to last for a continuous period of not less than 12 months"

Key Principles
- To be eligible for social security administration disability, the claimant must be totally disabled from gainful employment with an impairment that has lasted or is likely to last 12 months or more.
- When physicians determine disability, they must combine self-reports with objective medical information.
- Worker's compensation carriers are only responsible for work-related medical problems.
- Automobile insurance carriers are only responsible for injuries sustained during motor vehicle accidents.
- Apportionment is an attempt to allot causation among multiple medical sources.

Indications
- Not a standard component of clinical care
- Often requested by government, disability carrier, or employer

Contraindications
- None

Special Considerations
- An individual may have a serious impairment without a vocational disability.
- A mild impairment can have devastating vocational consequences.
- Disability is strongly dependent on the type of profession.
- Impairment ratings should not be done until individual has reached maximal medical improvement or for individuals with injuries that are not work-related.

Key Procedural Steps
- Diagnosis determination
- Determination of causation and apportionment
- Determination of need for further treatment
- Determination of impairment rating
- Physical capacity assessment
  - Ask patients to estimate their capacities.
  - Functional capacity evaluation
  - Functional restoration program
- Determination of ability to work by correlating patient's functional capacity with demands of the job

Anticipated Problems
- Clinical physicians may be unfamiliar with disability laws and may lack expertise in rating impairments.
- There is a possibility of deception on the part of the claimant.

Suggested Reading
Binder LM, Rohling ML. Money matters: A meta-analytic review of the effects of financial incentives on recovery after closed head injury. *Am J Psychiatr* 1996;153:7–10.

Intensity and Type of Rehabilitation Therapy

Description
- As with any medical or surgical intervention, rehabilitation services after TBI should be provided in the appropriate format, at the right intensity, for the optimal duration of time to have the greatest impact on the acute or chronic disability.

Key Principles
- TBI rehabilitation should be provided at the most effective intensity in the least restrictive environment available.
- A minimum of 3 hours of interdisciplinary therapy services is recommended for acute rehabilitation phase (2–8 weeks) after moderate and severe TBI for individuals who can participate. Individuals who cannot participate at this intensity or who have minimal disability should be delivered a less intensive service.
- Intensity and setting should be titrated based on progress on measurable outcomes.

Indications
- Any acute or chronic disability that may benefit from services
- All individuals with acute TBI who are functioning at the level of Rancho Los Amigos Scale III or higher are appropriate for intensive rehabilitation services.
- Individuals with severe TBI who are in a vegetative state are best treated with sensory stimulation in a medical setting.

Contraindications
- Inability to interact with the environment or learn/improve with services
- Medical instability that precludes active participation

Special Considerations
- Individualization of treatment settings to the unique needs of each patient is critical.

Key Procedural Steps
- Interdisciplinary treatment with active communication is critical.

Anticipated Problems
- The uniqueness of the skills set required and the intensity of the service mandate specialized TBI rehabilitation units.

Suggested Reading
Cifu DX, Kreutzer JS, Kolakowsky-Hayner SA, Marwitz JH, Englander J. The relationship between therapy intensity and rehabilitative outcomes after traumatic brain injury: A multicenter analysis. *Arch Phys Med Rehabil* 2003;84:1441–1448.

Outcome Assessment and Prediction

Description
- Outcome assessment is the use of standardized measures to quantify and qualify the current status of a patient with TBI.
- Outcome prediction is the use of historical, clinical, and neurophysiological data to approximate short- and long-term status.

Key Principles
- Outcome assessment is useful to objectively define a patient's status to determine current needs; provide feedback to patients, families, health care professionals and insurers; and determine the impact of acute care and rehabilitation interventions.
- Outcome prediction is used to provide input to patients, families, and health care professionals and insurers on probable short- and long-term future functioning so that planning may occur to provide for disability needs.

Indications
- Outcome assessment and prediction should be used for all individuals who sustain a TBI.

Contraindications
- Inexperience in outcome assessment may impact accuracy.
- Subjective bias or inexperience may adversely impact outcome prediction.

Special Considerations
- Early and aggressive medical and surgical stabilization is vital to achieve optimal recovery.
- All patients with moderate to severe TBI should be initially managed at a level I trauma center.
- Early rehabilitation delivered in an interdisciplinary setting at the maximal tolerated intensity (up to 3 hours/day) will optimize outcomes.
- Treatment environment should be the least restrictive possible that can safely manage a patient.
- Initial neurosurgical and trauma surgery management is vital for optimal outcomes.

- Interruptions in rehabilitation care due to medical or surgical issues will reduce short-term outcomes and may negatively impact long-term outcomes.

Key Procedural Steps
- Outcome assessment uses all aspects of clinical status to provide a comprehensive description of functioning. A number of measurement tools are used to describe physical, cognitive, behavioral, and functional abilities.
- Outcome prediction uses a weighted assessment of clinical functioning to develop short- and long-term predictions.
- The following negatively impacts short- and long-term outcome:
  - Prior disability, prior central nervous system, prior alcohol or substance abuse, age > 55 years at time of injury, severe brain injury, prolonged coma, prolonged posttraumatic amnesia, posttraumatic epilepsy, and limited or slow progression in therapy program, low level of arousal, poor cognitive functioning, particularly perceptual deficits, behavioral dysfunction, flaccidity, spasticity, and midline shift of > 5 mm on CT scan

Anticipated Problems
- Outcome prediction is usually based on population-based research, and therefore it may translate poorly to individuals.
- Acute deviations in functioning or in predicted outcome may suggest secondary diagnoses that may be treatable.

Helpful Hints
- Interdisciplinary input into outcome assessment and prediction will greatly enhance accuracy.

Suggested Reading
Mysiw WJ, Fugate LP, Clinchot DM. Assessment, early rehabilitation, and tertiary prevention. In: Zasler ND, Katz DI, Zafonte RD, eds. *Brain Injury Medicine*. New York: Demos; 2007:283–301.

Return to Sports

Key Principles

- For individuals with severe TBI, there should be stability of neurologic deficits and good performance with ADLs and mobility before consideration of return to sports.
- In severe TBI, there should be sufficient time between injury and return to sports to allow late recovery (6–12 months).

Indications

- All athletes who sustain TBI

Contraindications

- None

Special Considerations

- Decreased performance can increase risk of sports-related injury.
- Sports-related trauma may result in higher severity of injury due to underlying abnormalities.
- Second impact syndrome

Key Procedural Steps

Concussion Return-to-Play Guidelines

	First Concussion	Second Concussion	Third Concussion
Grade 1	No activity for 7 days if persistent symptoms RTP if asymptomatic	No activity for 4 weeks RTP only if asymptomatic for last 7 days	Terminate current season RTP after following season
Grade 2	No activity for 4 weeks RTP only if asymptomatic for last 7 days	Terminate current season RTP after following season	No activity for 1 year Ban contact sports RTP of noncontact sports in 1 year
Grade 3	No activity for 4 weeks RTP only if asymptomatic for last 7 days	No activity for 1 year Ban contact sports RTP of noncontact sports in 1 year	No activity for 1 year Ban contact sports RTP of noncontact sports in 1 year

RTP = return to play.

Suggested Reading

American Academy of Neurology. Practice parameter. The management of concussion in sports (summary statement). Report of the Quality Standards Subcommittee. *Neurol* 1997;48:581–585.

Return to Work

Description
- Many moderately to severely brain-injured individuals are unable to return to work, which leads to difficulties in psychosocial functioning.

Key Principles
- Brain-injured individuals may lack insight into cognitive and behavioral deficits, which may lead to resistance in vocational rehabilitation recommendations.
- Vocational rehabilitation should be a continuation of the overall rehabilitation process; resolution of all medical problems is not necessary.
- Success of vocational rehabilitation is dependent on severity of injury and the nature of medical and rehabilitative services provided after injury.
- Vocational rehabilitation should focus on ongoing cognitive, behavioral, social, and physical problems.

Indications
- All patients with TBI who are facing challenges with a return to productivity

Contraindications
- None

Special Considerations
- Individuals with brain injury may need extra supervision, more frequent rest breaks, or shorter work shifts.

Key Procedural Steps
- Vocational assessment takes into consideration the abilities and weaknesses of the brain-injured individual.
  - Vocational interest inventories
  - Assessment of perceptual-motor ability (ie, Purdue pegboard)
  - Objective tests for subskills
  - Work trials
- Vocational assessment also analyzes the relationship with the previous employer, the flexibility of the job for modification, and whether different forms of retraining are available.

Anticipated Problems
- Lack of insight into deficits
- Difficulty with self-direction
- Difficulty with adjusting behavior when problems arise
- Fatigue even after mild brain injury may be a significant limiting factor.

Helpful Hints
- Use a language-free vocational interest inventory consisting of pictures, if available, for the severely impaired individual.
- Work-hardening programs may help with fatigue but will fail to meet the needs of most traumatically brain-injured individuals.

Suggested Reading
Cifu DX, Keyser-Marcus L, Lopez E, et al. Acute predictors of return to work one year after traumatic brain injury: A multicenter analysis. *Arch Phys Med Rehabil* 1997;78:125–131.

Keyser-Marcus L, Bricout J, Wehman P, et al. Acute predictors of return to employment following traumatic brain injury: A longitudinal follow-up. *Arch Phys Med Rehabil* 2002;83:635–641.

Spasticity: Oral Medications to Treat

Drug	Mechanism of Action	Starting Dose	Maximum Dose	Advantage	Disadvantage
Dantrolene sodium (Dantrolene)	Believed to act directly on the sarcoplasmic reticulum by inhibiting calcium release	25 mg orally daily to start Then increase dose to 2 to 4× per day May then increase by 25 mg every 7 days	400 mg Doses beyond 200 mg not associated with increases in blood levels, but effect seen	Minimal cognitive side effects	Associated with hepatotoxicity
Baclofen (Lioresal)	Active at GABA-B receptor	5 mg orally three times daily	80 mg daily recommended Up to 160 mg daily may be considered	Can be given intrathecally for severe refractory spasticity	Sedating Memory dysfunction May not be as useful for upper extremity spasticity Abrupt withdrawal can be life threatening
Diazepam (Valium)	GABA-A receptor agonist	2 mg	40 mg	Useful for nighttime spasms	Sedating Impaired cognitive processing
Clonidine (Catapress)	α2 receptor agonist	0.1 mg daily	0.6 mg	Can help lower blood pressure in hypertensive patient	Dizziness Drowsiness Hypotension
Tizanidine (Zanaflex)	α2 receptor agonist	2–4 mg at bedtime	36 mg daily	Can help with both upper and lower extremity tone	Dizziness Drowsiness Hypotension Concomitant therapy with ciprofloxacin or fluvoxamine contraindicated
Gabapentin (Neurontin)	Mechanism unknown	300 mg orally three times daily Needs renal adjustment	3600 mg	Helps ameliorate neuropathic pain	Somnolence Dizziness Fatigue

Suggested Reading

Davidoff RA. Pharmacology of spasticity. *Neurol* 1978;28:46–51.

Index

Abducens nerve (cranial nerve VI) 66–67

Acute management, of TBI 165

Adrenal insufficiency 116

Affective lability. *See* Emotional lability

Agitation

    assessment scales 5

    medications to treat 166–167

    and restless behavior 26–27

Akinetic mutism 28–29

Anomic aphasia 30, 32

Anosmia

    cranial nerve deficits 60–61

Anterior attention network 34

Antidiuretic hormone, inappropriate

    neuroendocrine dysfunction 118

Anton syndrome. *See* Cortical blindness

Aphasia

    expressive (motor) 30–31, 32

    receptive (sensory) 30, 32–33

Apolipoprotein E4 biomarker

    dementia and TBI 74

Arousal level and attention

    assessment scales 10–11

Aspirin

    deep venous thrombosis (DVT) 73

Assessment scales

    agitation 5

    arousal level and attention 10–11

    balance and dizziness 6–7

    cognition 8

    concussion grading 9

    injury severity 9

    orientation 12–13

    postconcussion symptoms 14–15

    sleep 16

    smell 16

Ataxia 58

Attentional deficits, mild TBI 34–35

Attention Rating Scale 34

Balance and dizziness

    assessment scales 6–7

    diagnostic tests 17

Balance deficits 36–37

Behavioral physical examination 4

Bell palsy 63

Berg balance score 6–7

Bladder issues 38–39

Bladder urodynamics 18

Blast related injuries. *See* Combat related TBI

Bowel and bladder function

    diagnostic tests 18

Bowel issues 40–41

Bowel manometry 18

Brainstem Auditory Evoked Response 18

Brief Test of Attention 34

Broca aphasia. *See* Expressive (motor) aphasia

Burr hole. *See* Craniotomy

Caloric testing 17

Canalith repositioning maneuver 17

Central dysautonomia 42–43

Central sleep apnea (CSA) 108

Cerebrospinal fluid 134

Cervicogenic headache 126

CIMT. *See* Constraint induced movement therapy (CIMT)

Clonus 150–151

CNC. *See* Coma/Near Coma (CNC) scale

Cognition

    assessment scales 8

Cognitive deficits, of TBI 44–45

Cognitive physical examination 4

Color agnosia 160

Color imperception 160–161

Coma/Near Coma (CNC) scale 10

Combat related TBI 46–47

Complementary alternative medicine 168

Complex regional pain syndrome (CRPS)

    pain 122–123

Computer based cognitive therapy 169

Computerized posturography 6

Computerized tomography 21

Concentration Endurance Test 34

Concussion

    cumulative mild TBI 48–49

    grading, 9

    mild TBI 50–51

    postconcussive symptoms/syndrome (PCS) 52–53

    second impact syndrome 54

    sports 56–57

Conduction aphasia 30, 32

Conners' Continuous Performance Test 34

Constraint induced movement therapy (CIMT) 170–1719

Contrast Venography 23

Coordination deficits 58–59

Cortical blindness 160

Coup contracoup injury 20

Cranial nerve deficits

    anosmia 60–61

    face 62–63

Cranial nerve deficits—*Continued*
    head and neck 64–65
    ocular muscles 66–67
    special senses 68–69
Craniectomy 70–71
Cranioplasty 70–71
Craniotomy 70–71
CRPS *See* Complex regional pain syndrome (CRPS)
CSA. *See* Central sleep apnea (CSA)

DAI. *See* Diffuse axonal injury (DAI)
D-dimer blood test 23
Deep venous thrombosis (DVT) 72–73
Dementia and TBI 74–75
Dementia pugilistica 48
Depression 76–77
    medications to treat 172
Diabetes insipidus, central 116
Diagnostic tests
    balance and dizziness 17
    bowel and bladder function 18
    electrophysiologic evoked potentials 18–19
    neuroimaging findings in TBI 19–21
    neuroimaging techniques 21–22
    swallowing 22
    vascular 23
Diffuse axonal injury (DAI) 19, *20*
Disability determination 173
Disinhibition 78–79
Dix Hallpike maneuver 17
Dizziness 80–81
    and balance, 6–7, 17
DVT. *See* Deep venous thrombosis (DVT)
Dysarthria 82–83
Dysmetria 58
Dysphagia 84–85

EDH. *See* Epidural hematoma (EDH)
Electromyogram 18
Electronystagmography 17
Electrophysiologic evoked potentials
    diagnostic tests 18–19
Emotional lability 86–87
Enoxaparin
    deep venous thrombosis (DVT) 73
Epidural hematoma (EDH) 19
Epworth Sleepiness Scale 16
Executive function impairment 88–89
Expressive (motor) aphasia 30–31, 32

Facial agnosia 160
Facial nerve (cranial nerve VII) 62–63
FEES. *See* Fiberoptic endoscopic evaluation of swallowing (FEES)
Fiberoptic endoscopic evaluation of swallowing (FEES) 22
    limitations 84–85

Fondaparinux
    deep venous thrombosis (DVT) 73
Forced use therapy 170
Functional history 3

Gait (ambulation) dysfunction 90–91
Galveston Orientation and Amnesia Test (GOAT) 12
    modified 12–13
    for posttraumatic amnesia 134
Geriatric TBI 92–93
Gingko biloba 168
Glasgow Coma Score 9
Global aphasia 30, 32
Glossopharyngeal nerve (cranial nerve IX) 68
GOAT. *See* Galveston Orientation and
        Amnesia Test (GOAT)
Growth hormone deficiency 116

Headaches
    pain 126–127
Head and neck
    cranial nerve deficits 64–65
Hearing deficits 94–95
Hemiparesis 64, 65
    and hemiplegia 96–97
Heterotopic ossification 98–99
History 2–3
Hyperesthesia 100
Hyperprolactinemia 116
Hypertonia 150–151
Hypoarousal 102–103
Hypoesthesia and numbness 104
Hypoglossal nerve (cranial nerve XII) 64, 65
Hypothyroidism 116
Hypotonia and flaccidity 106–107

IEP. *See* Individual education plan (IEP)
Individual education plan (IEP) 128
Injury characteristics 2
Injury severity
    assessment scales 9
Insomnia 108–109
Intracerebral hematoma 20
Intraparenchymal hematoma. *See* Intracerebral hematoma

JFK Coma Recovery scale 10–11

Kava 168
Klüver Bucy syndrome 146

LIS. *See* Locked in syndrome (LIS)
LMWH *See* Low molecular weight heparin (LMWH)
Locked in syndrome (LIS) 110–111
Low molecular weight heparin (LMWH)
    deep venous thrombosis (DVT) 73

Magnetic resonance imaging (MRI) 21–22
MARS. *See* Moss Attention Rating Scale (MARS)
Medical exam, physical examination 4
Minimally conscious state 112–113
Modified barium swallow. *See* Videofluorography
Moss Attention Rating Scale (MARS) 11
MRI. *See* Magnetic resonance imaging (MRI)
Multiple Sleep Latency Test 16
Muscle trigger points 127
Musculoskeletal headache 126
Musculoskeletal physical examination 4

Narcolepsy 108
Neglect. *See* Spatial inattention, unilateral
Neuralgic head pain 126
Neuritic head pain 126, 127
Neurobehavioral Symptom Inventory 14–15
Neuroendocrine dysfunction 116–117
    antidiuretic hormone, inappropriate 118
Neurogenic dysphagia 84
Neuroimaging findings in TBI
    diagnostic tests 19–21
Neuroimaging techniques
    diagnostic tests 21–22
Neurolinguistic deficits, of TBI 120–121
Neurologic physical examination 4
Neuropathic pain 124, 127
Neuropsychological testing 8

Obstructive sleep apnea (OSA) 108
Ocular muscles
    cranial nerve deficits 66–67
Oculomotor nerve (cranial nerve III) 66–67
Olfactory nerve (cranial nerve I) 60–61
Optic nerve (cranial nerve II) 68
Orientation
    assessment scales 12–13
Orientation Group Monitoring System 13
Orthoptics 69
OSA. *See* Obstructive sleep apnea (OSA)
Outcome assessment 175
Outcome prediction 175

Paced Auditory Serial Addition Test 34
Pain 124–125
    complex regional pain syndrome (CRPS) 122–123
    headaches 126–127
    transmission 123
Paroxysmal autonomic instability with dystonia. *See* Central
    dysautonomia
Pathologic pain 124
PCS. *See* postconcussive symptoms/syndrome (PCS)
Pediatric TBI 128–129
Penetrating injuries 130–131
Physical examination 4

Physiologic pain 124
Picamilon 168
Piracetam 168
PLMS. *See* Posttraumatic hypersomnia, periodic limb
    movements in sleep (PLMS)
Polytrauma 124
Polysomnography 108
Positive emission tomography 22
Postconcussion symptoms
    assessment scales 14–15
Postconcussive symptoms/syndrome (PCS)
    concussion 52–53
Posterior attention network 34
Posttraumatic amnesia (PTA) 12, 13, 132–133
Posttraumatic hydrocephalus 134–135
Posttraumatic hypersomnia, periodic limb movements in sleep
    (PLMS) 108
Posttraumatic migraine 126, 127
Posttraumatic seizures (PTS) 136–137
Posttraumatic stress disorder 138–139
Posttraumatic tension headaches 126
Precocious puberty 116
Pressure sores 140–141
Pressure ulcers. *See* Pressure sores
Primary injury 130
Prophylaxis
    deep venous thrombosis (DVT) 73
Prosopagnosia. *See* Facial agnosia
PTA. *See* Posttraumatic amnesia (PTA)
PTS. *See* Posttraumatic seizures
Punch drunk syndrome 48
Pyritinol 168

Quadriparesis 142–143

Rancho Los Amigos Scale (RLAS), revised 8
Receptive (sensory) aphasia 30, 32–33
Rehabilitation therapy, intensity and type of 174
Rigidity 150–151
Rinne test 94
Rivermead Postconcussion Symptoms
    Questionnaire 14
RLAS. *See* Rancho Los Amigos Scale (RLAS), revised

SDH. *See* Subdural hematoma (SDH)
Secondary injury 130
Second impact syndrome
    concussion 54
Sexual dysfunction 146–147
Shaken baby syndrome 148–149
Sleep
    assessment scales 16
Smell
    assessment scales 16
Social history 3

Spasticity 150–151
  oral medications to treat 178
Spatial inattention, unilateral 114–115
Special senses
  cranial nerve deficits 68–69
Spinal accessory nerve (cranial
    nerve XI) 64, 65
Spinal cord and TBI
  dual disability 144–145
Sports
  concussion 56
  return to 176
St. John's wort (hypericum) 168
Subarachnoid hemorrhage 19
Subdural hematoma (SDH) 19
Swallowing
  diagnostic tests 22

THI. *See* Tinnitus Handicap
    Inventory (THI)
Timed Get Up and Go Test 6
Tinnitus 152–153
Tinnitus Handicap Inventory (THI) 6–7
Transcortical motor aphasia 30, 32
Transcortical sensory aphasia 30, 32
Transmission
  pain 123
Tremors 154–155
Trigeminal nerve (cranial nerve V) 62–63

Triple phase bone scan 23
Trochlear nerve (cranial nerve IV) 66–67

UFH *See* Unfractionated heparin (UFH)
Unfractionated heparin (UFH)
  deep venous thrombosis (DVT) 73
University of Pennsylvania Smell Identification Test 16

Vagus nerve (cranial nerve X) 64, 65
Valerian 168
Vascular diagnostic tests 23
Vegetative state, persistent 156–157
Venous ultrasound 23
Vestibulocochlear nerve (cranial nerve VIII) 68
Videofluorograph 22
Vigilance network 34
Vision deficits 158–159
Visual agnosia 160
Visual Evoked Potential 18
Visual perceptual deficits 160–161
Visual perceptual disorders 114
Vocational rehabilitation 177

Warfarin
  deep venous thrombosis (DVT) 73
Weber test 94
Wernicke aphasia. *See* Receptive (sensory) aphasia
Westmead PTA Scale 13
Work, return to 177